From ME to You, With Love

© Louise Harding 2014

ISBN: 978-1497569522

Lots of love,
Louise Harding
xxxx

This book is dedicated to anyone living with ME, and also to those people who continue to be there every step of the way... you know who you are.

I would like to thank the following people, without whom this book would never have happened.

To Rebeckah Rose for designing the cover.

To Jo Best, who has given me so much help and support, and who does so much for the 'Let's do it for ME!' campaign.

To Rob for being on my whole ME journey with me - and for letting me take over the computer!

To the very special people in my life who have given me so much love, support and encouragement in coping with my ME.

To my fellow sufferers and friends who continue to inspire me every day. I only hope that I can one day show half the level of bravery and strength that you do.

To everyone at Invest in ME and 'Let's Do it for ME!' for just being amazing.

To everyone who contributed to this book. Working with you on the 'Letters for Louise' project has been brilliant; you've helped me to strengthen old friendships and form new ones... and I am seriously grateful.

And finally to you, the reader, for helping us to be heard.

Contents

Dear World... 3

Dear Me... 70

Dear Professionals... 122

Dear Family... 180

Dear Friends... 225

Dear Sufferers... 249

Dear reader,

Firstly, thank you for reading this book and for taking the time to learn more about the condition myalgic encephalomyelitis (ME).

ME is defined by the World Health Organisation as a neurological illness. Many sufferers find that they develop it after some form of often quite normal virus or infection, and it affects many different systems in their bodies; the severity of people's conditions differ and can fluctuate over time, over months, weeks, from day-to-day or even hour-to-hour. Some people are affected mildly and may still be able to work, however their lives are still massively restricted and they miss out on doing a lot of things that a healthy person would take for granted. On the other end of the scale, someone who is very severely affected may spend months or years in bed, unable to care for themselves, feed themselves (so are tube-fed) or tolerate something even as simple as somebody else being in the room. There is currently no cure for ME.

The letters in this book come from sufferers of many different ages and with different severities of the illness, from all over the world and who have come from completely varied walks of life. However, what everyone has in common is that they have in some way become victims of misunderstanding or disbelief about their ME; they have come across people who have believed that it's 'all in your head' or that it's a case of 'mind over matter' (not helped by the fact that the illness has been labelled "Chronic Fatigue Syndrome" which wrongly suggests that sufferers are just tired). People with ME often find themselves constantly battling not only their illness, but also the views of those who believe a little bit of exercise and 'just getting on with it' will cure them, when in reality it has the opposite effect - it can make symptoms a lot worse. And instead of getting the compassion and support to get better that you would expect, many sufferers find themselves questioned as to why they don't want to get better or blamed for being ill. This is something that many people who have contributed to this book have found, and their stories represent a whole community of sufferers, who ultimately do not enjoy being ill and want nothing more than to get better. The letters that you are about to read are all completely real - as some contributors have chosen to remain anonymous, their names have been changed, but other than that each letter is completely honest and straight from the heart.

All profits from the sale of this book will go to the charity Invest in ME. They are a fantastic charity who work incredibly hard to raise awareness and fund biomedical research into ME. Despite there being a huge amount of evidence of a physical cause, there is no government funding into biomedical research because psychology has taken it on as 'their thing'. So Invest in ME's work is really important in funding research that would otherwise be left to one side, giving us a chance of finding a treatment or even a cure.

So thank you for taking an interest in our stories and becoming more aware about the reality of ME.

Louise Harding

Dear World...

To all readers of this book,

     For every letter you see here, there are countless others that ME sufferers wanted to write, but didn't have the cognitive or physical ability to make their voices heard. Please don't forget those of us who suffer in silence.

Thank you.

To anyone who wants to understand,

If I were to describe my illness to you, I would say it's like falling down a well. There are ledges, but if you move around too much you will fall further and further down. No-one tells you this though, so you keep trying to do the things you used to be able to until you hit the bottom of the well and there is nowhere left to fall.

You are on your own down there; it's painful, dark, and you're beyond exhausted. You try to think of a way out, but now even thinking shatters you. You cannot eat and everything hurts. It's quiet in the well, which is good because now you have fallen you are sensitive to noise. Everyone has left you because you are just out of their reach; you cannot participate like you could.

It takes you a few months, where all the people who love you make you a ladder and you begin to get ready to climb out. You take a step towards it, but you fall to the ground and have to rest for a few days. It takes you a year to get onto the first ledge. Remember - if you get too comfy and move too much, you'll fall, and all that work will be undone. You're on the ledge and you are exhausted; remember it took you a year to get here. You must rest for now.

When you and your body are ready, you take the next steps - this might be a few months on, or a year on. You have to go slowly so that you can sustain it - you want to get out of the well. So you climb, slowly, very slowly, but you're going up and up is good.

When you have rested at your next ledge you may carry on, but again it's going to take time - move too fast and you'll have to climb down to the level before, because you are ill - your body is ill.

So you're climbing and your arms hurt, your legs hurt, your back hurts, you have a headache, you feel dizzy and sick, but you must go down a few rungs to the ledge before and rest until you are ready.

By now, three years have gone by and you are half-way up. Well done - you have reached half-way, and this is incredible! There's a twist here. A reward.

You are still in the clutches of the well, but there is a world there - a world where you can do a bit more, you can walk a few metres - but only a few - you haven't walked for a long time remember.

You can go out with your best friend who is sat at the top of the well waiting for you, but you must not go far, because going too far could mean falling and falling could mean having this bit of life taken away.

You can have a shower now - you must sit down, but your mum will wash your hair. You see, your family and a few friends still haven't left you.

When your body can cope at this point, and this may take a year, you can start to climb again - maybe a little quicker this time; a step per week. You can now go out for three hours, but you must use a wheelchair. You may walk a few metres, but it will take longer to recover. You can have fun and it will maybe only take you a few weeks to recover from that outing.

I cannot comment on the next bit, for I have not yet been there, but I can see a little light at the top. It looks quite far away but I can see it, it's there, and it's waiting. I'm a little scared, because I haven't been in that world for four years, but one day my body will be ready and I will have recovered - whether that is a year from now or three, but I am going to the top. I still have to be careful because if I fall now I will lose all this once more, but I know now my limits. And if you are also suffering, you will learn yours too - you'll keep learning until you can wash your own hair, make your own food, wash your own clothes, work your own job and walk your own walk once more.

Lizzy Horn xxxx

Dear World,

> The truth about me with ME.

I AM STILL ME,

I am not the illness ME.

I seem to have turned into my illness, not a person. People no longer talk to me about normal, everyday things. Am I not a valued member of the world/ community/ family as I am ill and no longer able to work? I still am the person I was before ME, just I struggle at times. I get questioned from my husband - what time did you get up? Have you had some dinner? Have you been out? What are you doing? From friends: why can't you? Will you come? Why are you tired? Well we used to...

My personality is still within me somewhere, just I can struggle to be my usual self at times due to fatigue and pain. I do not mean to yawn when you talk to me, but I just can't help it at times. I may need to jiggle and move around - again, it does not mean I am not interested.

My intelligence is still within me somewhere, I still have the same qualifications as I had before the illness, just they can appeared masked for now.

Friends move on without you and leave you behind. After a time they stop calling and visiting as you say 'no sorry I can't, I am not up to it'. At times I can't even hold a conversation.

When I first got ME I was told 'you must learn to become selfish, you need to learn to put yourself first to be able to cope, to survive this illness'. I still toil over this; yes, it is kind of true but this does lead to further isolation and more barriers.

You go to speak to the GP to talk about new symptoms and they are often brushed under the carpet as 'just ME'. I was even asked if I felt my life was worth living and would I ever harm myself? I AM ME, NOT THE ILLNESS, yes - I may get down/ frustrated at times but I AM NOT DEPRESSED, I will not go away if I am drugged up with anti-depressants. After I first became ill and was examined it was put down to a functional illness; in other words, all in my head. The consultant even withdrew my painkillers. Luckily I was sent for a second opinion after a few months to another neurologist who believed me and carried out scans. My head pain (neuralgia) was treated and is still successfully treated - although my other pain is not, it's just my ME.

I have had to change life around, find new hobbies and interests that can be carried out within the boundaries of my illness. I have different capabilities, and maybe an altered outlook on life, but the main thing I would say is 'I AM ME, LOU, NOT THE ILLNESS'. I would still like to be talked to like your wife/ daughter/ friend/ member of the community.

Louise.

Dear people,

You often comment on my excitement for the smallest events and wonder how I manage to find the joy in the mundane. When you become so sick, you are left with no choice but to find small things incredible. The shade of blue the sky is, the time I saw a red kite over the garden, getting up the stairs alone, seeing a small child waving at you with a huge grin on its face. All of these things become major milestones in your life when your world has for such a long time consisted of four walls and nothing more.

This is just one way ME has changed my life, but maybe, just maybe it's not actually a change for the worse. Think about this when you next wonder why something is so exciting to me; don't get frustrated with me wanting to bathe in this glory. Don't huff and puff when I stop to take a photo of a tree; my memory is not what it was and these photos help me relive that joy I was feeling. Instead smile, and join me in the excitement of finding a ladybird or feeling the wind on my face.

Love from G xxxx

To those willing to hear my story,

It's October 2006 and I am standing in Chichester Festival Theatre having just received my 2:1 BA (Hons) degree for Teaching. I look into the crowd and see my parents, aunties and grandparents looking proudly on. I am an only child, and the only member of my family to go to university. I am excited about the future, having landed a job teaching Year 4 at my local primary school...

Flash forward to January 2014. I have just had to leave the job that I loved and worked hard for, for eight years. Did I not love teaching anymore? No. Had I moved away? No. The reason I left wasn't my choice... it was because of ME. Back in 2006 I had no idea about how these two letters would affect my life, but here I will share my story...

I was always a healthy child - good attendance at school and always outside playing imaginary games in the garden (often involving me tying my Roland Rat toy to the tree and rescuing him!) In March/ April 2005 I became ill with glandular fever. After that, I seemed to catch every bug going (including swine flu) and never felt 'right'. Despite numerous trips to the doctor, I kept being sent away, feeling more frustrated with each visit, and I felt the doctors just weren't listening to me.

It was only when I changed doctors in 2011 that finally the doctors started to listen. I explained all my symptoms and problems to my doctor who listened carefully and made lots of notes. He sent me for blood tests and spoke to me about the likelihood of me having something called ME - something I had never heard of before. He was in the process of referring me to the specialists when something happened to change my life.

On February 12th 2012 I went to work as normal. The day was going to be quite stressful as we had a county advisor coming in to do lesson observations (like a mock Ofsted inspection). It is very strange, but I can pinpoint the exact moment I felt my body go 'under attack'. I was in the middle of reading with a couple of children when I felt my whole body begin to ache (almost like I was being crushed under a steamroller!) and my head felt like it was going to explode. At playtime I popped a couple of paracetamol because I knew the county advisor was coming to see me after playtime. I somehow survived the observation and tried to carry on with my day.

However, after the end of the day bell rang I stumbled into the staff room, pale and grey and extremely dizzy. My friend Rachel took one look at me, went and collected my things and helped me to her car, telling me 'you are not driving home like this!' She kindly drove me home and helped me, along with my very concerned fiancé Marcus, upstairs and into bed. By now I felt extremely cold, yet actually had a raging fever. Rachel then went with Marcus to collect my car from the school grounds. When Marcus returned, he found me unresponsive in bed, quickly called an ambulance and then my parents to alert them to what had happened.

When I came to in hospital, I had a cannula in my arm and three worried faces looking at me. I had sticky pads all over me and despite all this my main worry was 'have I shaved my legs?!' I then had a rather traumatic episode of having another drip put into my left hand. I can only describe this pain as being something that I would imagine medieval torture to be. The bruising took forever to go down and even now, nearly a year later, my hand still feels tender to the touch. I vaguely remember a nurse talking to my mum and the nurse asking if I had ME, as all the things my mum was telling her about me suggested this.

I was let out of hospital much later that night. I then began three months of practically being bed-bound, feeling confused and pretty much useless. It felt like I had to learn things again - opening things, walking, stairs. All the time I was thinking how crazy it was - I used to ski, I used to play sports and it was only the previous summer I had done a road trip round America. In the summer I was trekking in the Grand Canyon, and now getting into and out of the bath wiped me out completely!

In May 2012 I was so stubborn and fed up I insisted on going back to work part-time. At first a good, structured plan was set up in accordance with Occupational Health suggestions, but as usual in my workplace things got shifted and my body could not cope. After more time off, I managed the last three days of term in July 2012.

I returned to work three non-consecutive days in September, once again with a Year 4 class. This worked well and I used my rest days to look after myself. However, my boss was keen for me to return to five full days and wasn't very nice to me. As the stress built up I decided that my health was far more important and I decided to leave my job. I was due to leave at the end of January 2014 but this was brought forward so I finished on the last day of term before Christmas.

So what now? For the time being, I shall be focusing on my health as I could feel the negative energy and stress from the work environment harming my already fragile body.

But I am not alone. My new journey, with ME as my travelling companion, includes my wonderful fiancé Marcus. He is always there for me, helping me do things, taking on extra work to support me and always runs me a lovely bubble bath to soothe my aching body. Thankfully he is strong enough to help me in and out and I jokingly liken it to Shamu the Whale at Sea World being launched into the pool! He has also been busy fundraising for Invest in ME as he is doing lots of running events including The Great South Run, Hastings Half Marathon and Brighton Marathon.

We have two miniature schnauzers called Kimble and Ellie who are a great comfort to me. Kimble can even tell if I am having a bad day and will climb up carefully to see me. Alas, Ellie hasn't seemed to catch onto this yet so charges at me and bounces up for a cuddle, then gives me apologetic licks when she realises I'm hurting. We also have two cats who love any excuse for an afternoon nap and to keep me warm.

Our families are constantly supporting us and I am also thankful to my ME friends. My dear friend Elaine from school also suffers from ME and even though she suffers greatly, she is always there for me, offering me advice and support. She is also extremely talented at crafting and has made me beautiful cards and bracelets. I have some skills to learn! She has also introduced me to a wonderful group of friends who are always there for me too. I hope one day we will all be well enough to meet face-to-face so I can tell them what great friends they are.

I am also fortunate to have a group of very dear friends, who look past my illness and see the old me. We can laugh and chat about anything and everything. When we were younger we used to go to Brighton on massive shopping trips. We recently went back to Brighton for a catch up. I felt nervous at first, worried that my ME would get in my way (I had rested for days prior to this trip but was still in pain), but my friends were so lovely and said they much preferred the constant sit down coffee breaks as 'we are getting old now' and prefer to sit down and have a good natter!

So this is me, with ME, facing new challenges and adventures every day, but surrounded by love and support. I hope one day a cure will be found and the daily pain will go away.

xx

Dear World,

'T is not too late to seek a newer world.
Push off, and sitting well in order smite
The sounding furrows; for my purpose holds
To sail beyond the sunset, and the baths
Of all the western stars, until I die.
It may be that the gulfs will wash us down:
It may be we shall touch the Happy Isles,
And see the great Achilles, whom we knew.
Tho' much is taken, much abides; and tho'
We are not now that strength which in old days
Moved Earth and Heaven, that which we are, we are;
One equal temper of heroic hearts,
Made weak by time and fate, but strong in will
To strive, to seek, to find, and not to yield.'

Tennyson wrote that (I think!). It made me reflect on what resolve my family and other loved ones wish that I had. But what could they see of it when will alone is not reversing the treachery that is ME?

I am not terribly eloquent, so you'll have to excuse my musings tonight.

I'm sorry that it seems to you that I've given up. I know no other way to keep the symptoms at bay - I am literally trapped in my own body that betrays me at every hurdle.

Sometimes, I see no way out from myself.

Despite my best efforts.

The physical pain is unbearable and I have borne it. The exhaustion is inexhaustible and I'm exhausted by that fact.

'Being' ceases to 'be' in any meaningful sense sometimes, yet I have no choice but to exist, awaiting its passage from me. At least in this world.

Often this seems the most pragmatic. But it lets me reflect on the blessing that it is to 'be' at all.

You claim my bed sucks me into an abyss, sometimes you see in me no more than my physically debilitated self. You identify me with this bed.

The bed that I despise. Or, as I once heard said, I try to unshackle myself from her bondage, yet the symptoms amplify and I'm filled with anxiety.

Your will clouds your vision. I wouldn't have it any other way, though; what right have I to ask you of anything else - you persist in feeding and sheltering me despite your will for me? How dare I?

Life speeds on ahead at a thundering pace, and is leaving me behind, and holding you back as you care for me whilst I lay, almost always limp, yet tense, in my bed.

I fear sometimes that your comments hold a great deal of truth. Yet the relentless illness, that strikes as such caprice in her manifested symptoms, are the only kernel to which I cling that convince me of what is real. Or at the very least, what seems real to me.

Though the fear of the next life haunts me - did I really fail to do my best to rid myself of this state?

Often I wonder what His will holds for me; and what vision I can manufacture of it. It's hard to know the mind of God.

Tell me what choices I have, and I will tell you that you have freed me.

From IS x

To those of you who have asked me what if feels like to have ME (and anybody else who is curious!)

What does it feel like to have ME? For me personally living with ME?

Well for starters, I feel intense head pain; severe, acute pain that painkillers cannot eliminate. It is severe enough to bring me to tears, to render me incapable of carrying out day-to-day activities. I feel it literally constantly.

I feel nausea; horrible waves of overwhelming sensations; it is severe enough to leave me curled up in a ball in bed, unable to move to avoid exacerbating it. I feel overwhelmed by the horrendous feeling of it, just waiting and wishing for the moment it eases.

I feel dizziness; I feel the room spinning around me on a daily basis. Of course the room I am in is doing no such thing, yet I feel it all the same. It can take away my sense of balance completely, so I am unable to walk at all without support.

I feel severe pain in my limbs; they squeeze tightly in on themselves in protest when I have used them too much (and 'too much' I can assure you is a very small amount).

I feel weakness in my limbs; they cannot work in the way everybody else's do, they just don't have the strength. I feel a fire burning in my throat every morning when I wake up. All too often, I feel a thick, cloudy fog in my brain stopping me from thinking clearly. I cannot speak, type, write, listen, or comprehend without a huge amount of focus and concentration which is so often utterly beyond me.

And lastly I feel exhaustion which I have left until the end to describe as it is the hardest for a non-ME sufferer to make sense of. Before becoming ill, I could count on one hand the number of times I had ever felt the levels of exhaustion which I now feel; every. Single. Day.

The exhaustion feels like powerful tidal waves surging over me. They cannot be escaped, however hard I might try. I feel the ME exhaustion turn my body into stone, so that every movement is a trying task; lifting a limb is like lifting rocks. I feel the ME exhaustion slowing down my mind, I feel it tug at my eyelids so that it is a desperate battle to keep my eyes open. I feel it overwhelm my senses with fatigue and drowsiness, I feel it enticing, compelling, demanding me to sleep. However, when I do sleep, ME will not allow that sleep to be refreshing, so that it can continue its cruel cycle once more, when I awake as tired as when I succumbed to sleep.

...all of these symptoms I feel come and go, in varying combinations and varying severity, so that some days/hours are better than others - but I am never without at least one and rarely without two or more.

...but none of this tells you what it really, truly feels like to have ME. The emotional repercussions of those physical feelings are as bad to live with as the physical symptoms themselves. I feel a myriad of thoughts and feelings after so long living with ME.

I feel I am a failure. I feel I have achieved so little with my life. I feel scared of the future; I want to get a degree, a career, a family of my own, and yet how can I, stuck in the grip of ME? I feel isolated. I feel lonely. I feel left behind. I feel a disappointment to my family. I feel a burden. I feel anger. I feel despair. I feel sadness. I feel it is unfair. I feel so very tired of being so very ill for so very long. And I could go on.

Yet every coin has two sides.

I feel the strength of the wonderful people I have met as a result of living with ME. Their strength, courage and determination shine through to me, through telephone lines, through text messages, through emails, through Facebook, to reach me and to inspire me. I feel a sense of community and acceptance within the ME world. I feel determined to live my life to the fullest I am able. I feel hope that one day I will recover. I feel lucky to have such wonderful friends and family. I feel grateful for everything good in my life of which there is so much. I feel proud of myself for getting through every tough day.

But most of all I feel that yes, I have been through a very difficult seven years, facing deteriorating health, which has been exhausting both mentally and physically, but I feel due to that I have become a stronger person, a more empathetic person, a calmer person, a more thoughtful person, a more determined person, a kinder person, ultimately a better person

So there you have it - that is what it feels like to be me with ME.

xx

To anyone who wants to know what having ME is like,

      I can see the darkness surrounding me as I lie awake, with only the light from the parts the blackout blind doesn't cover for company; such is the fate of this night's insomnia.

But whilst the night grows old and morning comes to fruition, I feel the wash of sleep come over me.

When I wake again it is light, and through bleary gaze I know it's time to get up.

I hear people going to work and wish I was with them, that that commute was mine, that that job was mine to nurture and be rewarded for.

Instead, crawling to the edge of the bed, my joints let me make progress to the scene of breakfast.

Already I feel that half the day has been lived as I will myself to concentrate and push through the deadening weariness that consumes my body whole.

I glance at the to-do list and realise the amount of energy I have doesn't equate to the amount needing to be done.

So things become prioritised, and only those things that are critical make the final cut.

How I'd wish to do them all and know that relief of reaching the final task.

Once the daily ablutions of the day are complete, the sofa calls to me its lonesome song.

I'd planned to go out today, do the exercise I'd been promising myself, but I know that that day is not today.

Today is about stealing time from a body that knows nothing about time, only that this doesn't function in the normal nine-to-five grind.

It's awful to think of the contradictory conflict that home is your prison, but also where you want to be.

How in turn you long for pillow and duvet, yet yearn for work and lunch.

And so the day progresses, trying not to fall asleep in meals, and to pay attention to conversations that surround you, and hope the pain is manageable.

But so often it's about hope, hope that this day will be the last of this relapse, that tomorrow will be different, will be better; but as the day grows old, the hope fades and before long you yearn for stillness and rest, and night-time is once more.

Xx

To journalists and others who work in the media,

In years to come - hopefully not many - people will look back with utter disbelief and perplexity at the way people with ME are treated. You in the media world could have a major role to play in highlighting and challenging these great injustices. If you want to make a real difference in the world, here is a golden opportunity; please, please take it. If you want to create a sensational, fascinating, life-changing piece, this is a great story to cover. Devastating levels of suffering; the impact on families and carers, the huge cost to society, widespread medical neglect and abuse, heroic efforts by patients and their families to survive and also to raise awareness and funds for research, psychiatrists ignoring over fifty years of quality scientific research in order to further their own vested interests by making false claims about a severe neurological disease, leading to children being taken from their parents and multiple unjust incarcerations in psychiatric units; and the list goes on. There is plenty of material here and many different angles you could cover.

Did you know that ME has many clinical similarities with MS? Yet how many MS patients are denied any form of appropriate care and treatment - an almost universal experience for people with ME? How many MS patients have the experience - that is all too common for people with ME - of being met with derision, scorn, ignorance, misunderstanding and disbelief by their doctors, employers, families and friends? How many people with MS would have the experience that I, a person with ME, did; of asking my purported 'specialist' for advice about symptom management but being told 'no', that's not something they can offer - and I was then given a poem about loving myself as I am? I then fought for about four months to even speak to the consultant (who I've never been allowed to have contact with), only to be eventually told that he can't see me because I am housebound and he doesn't have funding for home visits or telephone calls. But I'm one of the lucky ones - at least I haven't been forced into undergoing 'therapies' (such as GET - Graded Exercise Therapy) which have been proven to make people with ME worse - but far too many people have been forced into it.

This appalling situation must not be allowed to continue unchecked and in silence. ME is a devastating disease that ruins lives - but the way we are treated takes the suffering to a whole new and unnecessary level. Please, journalists and others who work in the media, please speak up for us. People with ME are brave warriors who fight on just to survive, just to do basic things that other people take for granted. We are poles apart from the psychiatric lobby's description of us as malingering, lazy and deconditioned. We will continue to fight, we will continue to raise our voices to try to be heard - and you have the power to make a huge difference in our fight. Please don't be yet another one who ignores us.

Thank you.

A desperate plea to the world,

I was thirteen years old when my world fell apart. I fell ill with a horrendous illness, which has tortured me every second of every day since. Year after year I have been getting worse and worse, losing my ability to walk, to stand, to sit, to use my arms or legs, to read, to watch TV, to tolerate any sound. I have lost all my teenage years and my twenties to this monstrous illness. I have lost my ability to study, to work, to have a family or a social life. I have lost everything I love and cherish to this illness. It has prevented me from living or leaving any mark in this world. I'm afraid I will die with nobody, except my closest family, even knowing I ever existed. The name of this illness is myalgic encephalomyelitis, also known as ME.

Even the slightest activity (such as lifting a glass of water) causes extreme weakness and paralysis, which makes me unable to move my arms or legs. On bad days I am too weak to change position in bed, speak or chew food. I suffer with bedsores as a consequence of not being able to change position. When my noise sensitivity is at its worst, even the slightest sound of a whisper causes extreme pain throughout my spine, neck and body. These phases of complete intolerance to sound can last for a year at a time. I have to spend most of the time lying in complete darkness and silence, too weak to move. Still, there are ME patients who are even more ill than I am.

I am bed-bound and need as much help as a tetraplegic. Without the 24/ 7 help from my family I wouldn't stay alive. Because of the complete ignorance amongst doctors about ME, I am left without any medical help. Just like so many others with severe ME, I have been left to rot in my own bed, without even the most basic health care. I am too sick to even visit a doctor and much too sick for a hospital, since all sound, light, stimuli and activity causes my condition to deteriorate further.

I have been humiliated and abused by doctors and forced into 'treatments' which have damaged my health further. The most damaging treatment being forced upon us is Graded Exercise Therapy, which causes permanent and severe damage to persons with ME. All this because of a complete ignorance amongst the medical establishment about the true nature of ME, where even minimal activity causes a significant and often permanent worsening of the condition. There seems to be close to no knowledge at all about the serious and potentially fatal neurological illness that ME is. ME is constantly lumped together with various fatigue-conditions, which means research isn't getting anywhere and hence no hope of a treatment either. There is no research being done on severe ME and there are no treatments available, nothing to stop the progression of this merciless illness.

This needs to change! So many young people, like myself, are losing their whole lives to this illness. We are too ill to fight. We are too ill to scream and shout and make ourselves heard. Please fight for us! Please let doctors, researchers and governments know about the reality of true ME. Please don't let us die in vain, fading away in dark and silent rooms, isolated from the whole world.

Maria

To anyone who thinks I'm exaggerating, or making this all up,

Let me take you back to 2011. I've been lying in bed for two weeks pretty much solidly, after a really awful, long (weeks rather than days) hospital stay. I've got carers coming in three times a day. I can just about walk from my bed to the edge of my room with a walking frame, a lot of help, and an awful amount of effort. But that can only happen every few days because it knocks me back massively. Today, however, it's different. Something exciting is happening. I'm actually going out! OK it's only to a hospital appointment, but I haven't left my bedroom for two weeks. My carer is getting me dressed, and I realise that this is the first time I've worn shoes in two months. This appointment is going to make me feel seriously ill in the coming days and weeks, but at the moment I'm not that bothered. I've got an ambulance coming to take me down the stairs and to the hospital, then they'll be taking me home, carrying me upstairs again and I'll be back in bed. But I'll have been out, and at the moment that's all that matters. How old am I? You'd probably guess in my late seventies, eighties or even nineties. No, I'm twenty-two.

Fast forward to very recently, to 2013. Luckily, I'm not severely affected by ME anymore. I'm working and am now a home owner, and on the surface I'm completely fine. Some people know that I have ME, some don't. Some people know how ill I've been in the past, some don't. I try and keep it all as low key as possible. But recently I've been struggling to do that, to keep it under wraps, because I am seriously beginning to suffer and I am scared. Even though I've had ME for many years, the memories of my spell being a severe sufferer still haunt me. I don't quite know how I got through that spell and I'm really worried that if I go back there, this time, I won't get through it. On the surface, at work, I'm managing to keep it together... just. But when I get home I can't hold it in anymore, can't hold it all together. I feel so drained that all I can do is sit at the bottom of the stairs and cry because I can't get up. I feel pain in every single muscle that is so intense it makes me physically sick. Sometimes it's so awful to move that I only just get to the loo in time. I feel dizzy, sick, faint... but above all, scared. I try and get an early night to try and be as strong as possible the day after, but often I'm feeling so awful I can only sleep after taking a lot of very strong drugs, which I know will leave me feeling groggy in the morning - but it's my only hope of sleep.

All of that, I can cope with because I've experienced a lot worse in my time. But what I am really finding difficult is the atmosphere I'm feeling from some of the people I'm around. Not all, just a few... but it's really hurting. They haven't said anything to me, but I've sensed that they're getting fed up of me. I don't go out with them, I moan, I need to just get over it, I look fine, I'm just looking for an excuse because I'm actually pretty rubbish at what I do, I just like getting attention, I just keep going on and on... but the thing is, the really frustrating, irritating thing, is that none of that is true. I don't like the attention that ME brings, I despise it. I despise being different. I would give anything to go out. I feel like screaming, 'WHY CAN'T YOU GET IT?!?!' But if I do, that'll just be playing up to what they think of me.

Even now, right here in 2014, sometimes, trying to fight against people's attitudes is so much worse than the ME itself. You feel so isolated, unable to speak out. People only see what they want to see. I'm not a liar, I'm not exaggerating. I don't want this illness; I'm not trying to look for an excuse. People don't know what I'm like out of the 'public eye' as it were because I'd like to think that I do a pretty good job of disguising the ME. Just because I'm not severely affected anymore, it doesn't mean that I don't suffer.

I'm lucky because there are people around me who are just incredible. They listen and they understand. They take the time to talk to me, they look after me when I'm having a bad day and most of all they believe me. And to those people, I want to say thank you so much because you make the fight worthwhile. You've shown me that I am worth something and I'm determined to find a way of succeeding because of you. To you, I am me, not ME.

In the future, I'd love to see a treatment that can help me to cope a little bit better, or even a cure. But first of all I'd love to see people listen and take on board what life is like for those of us with ME. I'd like to feel able to talk to someone about what ME is and how it affects me, and to not worry that they're thinking 'oh yeah...' as I'm speaking. I'd like to stop being ashamed of my illness.

Believe me, this is not the life I chose at twenty-four years old. It's not the life I want. But I hope it's still a life that I can look back at in years to come and be proud of... and make something good come out of it all.

All I ask is if you don't believe that ME sufferers are as ill as they say they are, please keep it to yourself. Because trust me, there is a lot that we keep to ourselves!

Xxxx

To anyone who doesn't understand,

Try to understand how tired I am feeling
Try to understand why I may not look my best
Try to understand that inside I am reeling
Try to understand that I really have to rest

Try to understand I hurt more than I share with you
Try to understand my thoughts are often hazy
Try to understand I can't live my life like you do
Try to understand it's not because I'm lazy

Try to understand I need you on my side
Try to understand that every day I fight
Try to understand there is so much I try to hide
Try to understand I am not like this out of spite

Try to understand I don't want to let you down
Try to understand I am interested in what you say
Try to understand how much it takes to meet you in town
Try to understand my challenges every day

Try to understand I wish I could say I'm fine
Try to understand I am still the same person
Try to understand the suffering is mine
Try to understand alone I carry this burden

Try to understand it's still me in here
Try to understand when I can't get out of bed
Try to understand I live in fear
Try to understand why I sometimes wish that I was dead

Try to understand the answers are not there
Try to understand that the doctors cannot cure me
Try to understand that it's hard to show you that I care
Try to understand that this is ME.

Xxxx

An open letter to all who will read it...

    Life sucks sometimes!

I'm so alone; my illness makes me have to shut everyone out. People come and go but mostly go, leaving me stuck in the house, lying in bed whether I'm ill or not. No-one takes the time to read into my illness or takes the time to listen to me. The nature of ME means I can't predict my health, I have to cancel last minute whether I like it or not and that leaves me constantly letting people down - and that's exactly why they leave. No-one wants a friend who can't reply to texts or emails because they're too tired, no-one wants someone who can't go out or make plans with them because they're constantly ill. Who would want to be close to me? I understand it, I really do but it doesn't stop it hurting when I'm alone and watching others enjoy their lives with friends, partying and having the fun they're meant to be having, going to the prom and having the education I dream of.

You never know what you have until it's gone. Simple everyday things become so hard to manage; washing, walking, getting drinks, going to the bathroom. It's all too much for me sometimes and it's the worst feeling in the world not even being able to do the most basic of tasks for yourself. I have a wheelchair and crutches; it sounds like nothing but it's so much more than it sounds. I suffer from anxiety and depression, I feel sick, shaky and just so horrible out in public. I struggle with confidence anyway and dislike the way I look so much; it's hard to look past the anxious feelings I get when I go out in my wheelchair or crutches, since there's so much contributing to it.

I just feel so alone and unwanted. I have only one true friend and he's amazing but I feel like I have no-one else. My boyfriend's a big part of my life also and it helps me so much. I just wish I had the friendship groups other girls my age have.

I needed to rant about how I feel; bottling it up inside is so horrible but no-one understands or knows how to help.

My life isn't full of pain, loneliness and misery – although that is a big part of it. I have good days where I can enjoy my photography and my family, friends and boyfriend's company and manage small activities, but it is SO limited and SO hard, always with payback. This is just something that haunts me every day of my life living with ME and I wanted to share it with you.

xxx

Dear readers,

Alive but not living:

Alive but not living
My life has lost meaning
I feel like I'm dreaming
And want to start screaming
I think of life missing
And go into grieving
There comes some accepting
Yet I can't help crying
Part of me is changing
There is no denying
For sure I'm not lying
Believe me I'm trying
So hard to keep breathing
Carry on believing
Not to give up hoping
For a cure I'm praying
How I hate this feeling
It's all so frustrating
I try to keep smiling
But it's so depressing
Survive but not living
So tired of fighting
Feel no-one is helping
I'm left slowly dying.

© 2013 Ros Lemarchand

To those who dismiss ME as depression,

>   Depression versus ME.

You say I'm just depressed, that is why I have these symptoms? You say that all I need is fresh air and exercise? That being in one room, in one bed, has made my symptoms arise. The lack of light, lack of movement, and the isolation... IMMOBILITY syndrome... it was bound to happen after all. No-one can shut themselves away and not cause themselves physical and psychological damage, surely?

Let me enlighten you, let me explain. Depression and ME, the one and the same? No, I think not.

I have had both. Extreme depression as a teenager, where I couldn't bear sunlight, to wear colour, to be with another human being. A life of greyness, dullness, where nothing mattered or moved me. Lethargy, lack of interest in things future, present, and past. Not wanting to exist. My bedroom and my cat, they were my world and I was happy for it to be so small.

Now severe ME as an adult. Now forced into one room, devastation at the smallness of my world, frustration that I cannot move, create, discover... due to my body not responding, my mind not working, battling fatigue, pain, and weakness. Fear, loss of control, ashamed, lack of dignity. Anger at the disbelief and criticism.

Yes, I've wanted to cease to exist with severe ME, but only because I want the horror to end, the unbearable, endless suffering. But, if there was a choice, I would rather get well than die. With depression I couldn't see beyond that illness, beyond that world, nor did I want to. With ME I choose to live, despite the horror. With ME I fight, fight, fight!

Now I have both, but the depression is as a RESULT of the ME. For twelve years of being physically consumed by illness

I warded off that black mind-set, always using every ounce of my precious energy to plan, dream of and create my recovery. Even paralysis, the terror, the trauma, the dispiriting comments from others didn't put me back into depression.

And now, even though I am recovered to the point of being able to wash myself, feed myself and walk a few steps a day, what has brought on depression is FRUSTRATION. And the more I recover the more frustrated I get. The world is there for me but I cannot enter.

So the depression with ME, they can go hand in hand, the one revolving round the other at times, and one could say the depression with ME is a depression of its own. One of despair, driven by being motivated and willing yet unable in the flesh.

However, whatever the cause, depression and ME, they are worlds apart and should NEVER be confused. X

Dear DWP (Department of Work and Pensions),

I would just like to tell you that although you don't know me at all, you have had a massive impact on my life.

Over twenty years we have had an acquaintance, and a few battles along the way. I have won most of those, which has helped; however, over the last year and a half as much as I've fought, I don't have any more energy left to fight. You have won, you have left me with nothing.

I have had government funded solicitors which have been absolutely useless. I have been to all agencies that I can, however all to no avail.

Over the eighteen months, I have had a very strong case; rock solid I thought, but in the end I don't think it mattered what I did or said, I feel it's prejudiced.

You don't seem to understand that I can get work, I've been offered many jobs; I've proved that to you, but it just doesn't sink in. I am ill; that's why I can't work. Why don't you understand that I have qualifications that get me many offers of, in some cases, very reasonable pay? Why would I have the qualifications if I didn't want to work?

I have been offered jobs in the USA, Pakistan and many places around the UK. I have given you this info for verification, yet you still think I would rather be housebound almost, living off your measly amount, when I could earn so much more; your rationale beggars belief.

N.

To the state benefits system of the UK,

>   I'm no sponger!

Since 2001, since this illness began, I've filled out your forms and answered your questions. Reams of paperwork, again and again. Such silly questions too - can I set an alarm clock? Can I lift an empty cardboard box? Can I lift my hand as if to put a pen in my top pocket? I can actually do all three in a strong moment, not that I have pockets in my nightie. Maybe I could get a job as a Putting-a-Pen-in-a-Top-Pocketer.

But can I walk? No. Am I always able to speak and understand? No. Can I guarantee I'm not going to vomit/ collapse/ shake uncontrollably/ pass out/ cry with pain...? No. Seriously, would you employ me?

And your medicals. Yes I might look OK, yes I might be able to raise my arm, but ask me to raise it more than a few times and you'll be picking me up off the floor. Having me in bed for weeks. Not that you'll see that. You don't see us ME'ers once we are home again. Every task an Olympic challenge, with severe symptom punishment as a consequence.

Yet it's not just me. Now I am bedridden you can't really argue with that, although you've tried, but what about the others? My fellow sufferers, those who aren't as ill as me but still so unbearably unwell. Their lives ripped apart, dominated by this horrendous condition.

As if the suffering isn't enough, the torturous, unbelievable symptoms, you then tell us we exaggerate, invent, are frauds. I'm not quite sure you understand the magnitude and devastation of being labelled a sponger. The terrifying fear that our money will be stopped, of being made destitute, the horror of having to find work when we feel on our death bed.

Us with ME, we are the perfectionist personalities, the driven achievers. You should be weeping that you don't have us well enough to work. You should be striving for a cure, desperate not to waste such talent, lose out on our contribution to society.

Believe me, if we weren't such, we would be dead a long time ago, having given up on our lives, on any chance of better days. Which perhaps we have in a way sometimes, but only because you beat it into us that this is all in our mind, that we are slackers, are cheats. (Funny how we aren't allowed to give blood. We are making all these symptoms up of course, but just in case it's not psychiatric...)

You call in the psychiatrists; you try to convince us we are anything but physically ill. Then you give us the ME clinics. 'Experts' in the field, those who have never experienced the misery of ME, full of NHS wisdom. You give us Graded Exercise Therapy, Cognitive Behaviour Therapy. Not that you ask us for our opinion of what might these treatments be doing to us. NICE guidelines, PACE trial, treatments made up by those who believe we can push ourselves well over time. Extending our physical boundaries, creating stamina, as if we were recovering from a sprained knee.

Half-hearted, feeble attempts fed by inaccurate information. I've had to pay many pounds for my own private treatment, saving the measly pennies you throw at me, surviving on hand-outs. Treatment which actually helps a bit, makes sense, put together by other recovered patients, but of which you won't listen to, not wanting to overturn your set-in-stone mind-set.

And then there is the funding. Over a year I waited for approval to go into hospital when I was so ill I couldn't move. The only two beds in the country dedicated to ME. On a psychiatric ward. In the end I declined your offer. I discovered it wasn't worth the wait.

I've written to my MP about you, told on you. Not that I've had a response, but at least I've officially aired my upset. For all the good it would do. And was that you sitting outside my home, watching, waiting to see if I would climb ladders in the driveway, lift weights, do somersaults? I bet you were bored.

Us with ME, we go it alone, en masse, fighting for recognition, for acceptance, to be taken seriously. Our own fundraisers, educating doctors, encouraging and advising each other. A voice from indoors, under duvets, shouting over the internet.

Not that I'm ungrateful for hard-working tax payer's money, truly I am, and I use it wisely, but please don't make me beg for it. I am hard-working, eager to please and only wish you would see that within me.

MB

To the Governing Bodies World-Wide,

Please tell me how can you sit in your high raise offices with comfortable high-back leather chairs sat around a polished oak table, with fresh coffee and snacks and decide file-by-file who gets a treatment and who doesn't? What in this world are you thinking? How can you sleep with yourself at night time?

All evidence points to these illnesses, ME, Lyme's, GWS and others being physical diseases, and you have mountains of data on patients who you are allowing to suffer daily and do nothing. Where is your compassion for a human life? Who made you God?

Why are you allowing this tyranny to continue, day after day? Why have you rendered the doctors helpless? Why put a professional in the position of deciding between their livelihood, career and family or helping the sufferers?

You have the data and you have the information, yet you choose to ignore the pain and suffering; I don't know how a person could do this. Does it make it better that there are several of you deciding this fate, that if you are all in argument then you personally are not to blame?

You know if this is contagious, yet you allow patients to have no idea of what the risks are, of what this disease is. You allow patients to roam around increasing the risk-factor, possibly. You know it comes in outbreaks. Surely you are a body of people that is supposed to protect the health of the world? When did that get pushed aside?

Why do you allow the misinformation that this is a mental illness - don't you think the sufferer is suffering enough with the attitude of medical professionals? Then you add this to our plate, and then you wonder why we are getting sicker. Or you falsify figures to suit what you want the public to know, or mess with reports so it doesn't look so bad.

Where-oh-where did human decency, compassion, understanding, or JUSTICE go in this world? Seriously, you hold the power and you are abusing it, and still you go home to your suburban homes, in your luxury cars, and sit around a dining table with your family and eat and laugh. I have no clue how you can do this, knowing what you know. Me, I'd be ashamed and I wouldn't be able to get the words I've seen in patient files out of my mind - it would haunt me forever.

I am a follower of Jesus, and do you think that you will go unpunished for these deeds? Look back in history of all that have been before who used these tactics on people, Ruhollah Khomeini, Idi Amin Dada, Pol Pot, Adolf Hitler and Josef Stalin. I personally put you in with these people - that is how strongly I feel. I am wondering who needs the psychiatrist, the ones you push the sufferers towards.

Ms. T

Dear World,

>'Silence is not golden'.

I look back over the many, many years and see how I have struggled, and I weep in silence. I am reminded daily of why 'in silence'! My culture, my faith, my friends and even family have taught me very implicitly and have been the voice in my head whispering 'if you stop now, if you sleep too much, if you voice a complaint even about pain, you are a lazy wife, a lazy mother and a woman without trust in God!'

So in essence what it all came down to was this; 'you are weak!' So I fought every moment extra hard when I was facing my battle and my fatigue, pain, etc. was out of remission due to unfortunate events which led to stress. I pushed so hard and made every excuse under the sun as to why I was sleeping so much, why I was suffering headaches to the point of looking down the toilet bowel once too often, why I isolated myself, made dates with friends and became so good at finding reasons to cancel almost every time and soon enough they became frustrated with me. I will never forget the day my husband (who was oblivious about my struggle as I had not been formally diagnosed, but was aware that things were not quite the way they should be) discussed with me the financial need for both of us to work. I remember the exact spot I was standing in two years ago and my thought was 'how will I cope, how will I do this?' The fear gripped my heart - but once again, 'silence'.

I started my full-time employment in a field that I studied for. I love my work and always say I was born to do this. I work in Mental Health as a Community Support Worker. In my first year I struggled so hard each day with all the symptoms, and once again pushed myself harder than before through the exhaustion and pain etc. And made excuses once again when people asked me why I looked ill. It reached a point where I ended up in hospital having an emergency blood transfusion.

Over the following months my situation worsened with other health issues and I lessened my work hours from five days (which nearly killed me) to four days. Before long the doctor had declared me unfit to work for a month. I am on this last week of the month. Once again the fear strikes me (me, who has handled adversity to the hilt and back and walks fearlessly). The fear is of the unknown again, of not being able to get past the thought of judgment of the lack of understanding on people's part. The look of 'doubt' on people's faces (the handful) when I share my story. My family's confusion as to what this is all exactly about. Can I blame them? How can I blame them if they have not been educated? If there is not highlighting of this disease, of this chronic illness this wife and mother has lived with for so many years - how can they understand? How can they overcome their fear? I feel as sad for them as I do for myself.

In a world where modern technology reigns supreme, in a country where medical intervention is deemed superior, then why do I still have these questions? Why do I live stigmatised? I need answers as much as my fellow sufferers do. Our recovery journey has to have answers so that we can continue freely with our healing.

Yours,

Nola

Dear World, or whomever this is suitable for!

I get so angry with you sometimes; why have you given me this thing that I don't understand, that the world doesn't seem to understand? I want to know what it is that makes me feel this way, I want to be able to slap it across the face and say 'how dare you! What gave you the right to do this to me?! Who the hell do you think you are?!'

There is no point in being angry with you though is there? There is no point in trying to find answers that just aren't there. I'm in the situation I'm in because I'm in it, and for the moment I can't change it.

I will fight this - don't think for a second world I won't! I'm going to keep on enjoying my life, even though I will pay for it physically when I do. I will continue to love all those around me who show me such boundless support, and I will ignore those that don't.

This is an opportunity, I will not let this destroy my life, I will only let it point me in a new direction.

So yeah, sometimes world or whoever the hell this should be directed at, I cry; so what the hell does that matter? Most of the time, I stay strong and I try not to let ME define me.

You go annoy somebody else; I've had enough of you now.

Karen

To readers; my thoughts on a discharge 'care plan' for someone with an unrecognised physical illness, after three years of psychological torture,

Some people have been asking me about what plans are being put in place to support me in my home when the NHS washes its hands of me on January 21st. The short answer is, so far, nothing; but a month ago, I put down some thoughts for the organisation that is ostensibly going to be helping me. These notes may help explain a situation that may be quite common to people cut down by ME, and similar 'invisible' illnesses:

One of the reasons I was keen to have xxxxxxx involved, is that I do not have any recent experience of living on my own; and have no experience of doing so as a mostly bed-bound disabled person with no friends, and no hope of getting better thanks to having been blacklisted and turned away by the NHS. I did live alone for most of my life and was pretty much self-sufficient, as I could turn my hand to almost anything that needed to be done. This ability, however, meant that there were certain skills I did not learn - how to earn money, for one, and how to spend it, for another! It meant that I never had to think about what to do next, because there was always something crying out to be done - always something that had to be made, maintained, or repaired, or something that someone else wanted me to help them with. Most of my 'friends' were people I fixed things for, or got involved with environmental or rights campaigns with, so the concept of being helped is quite alien to me and I need xxxxxxx's experience to suggest what my needs may be.

Thus, my well-being and livelihood, and my reason to exist, were all dependent on remaining healthy - which, through my interest in fitness and healthy eating, I had reason to think I would do. Looks pretty dumb now! With my health and my 'friends' gone, I have to learn how to live from scratch as a severely disabled person, which is completely against my nature; especially as I am still of the opinion that this 'disability' is an illness that could be remedied if only the NHS would take it seriously and make a real effort to find out what it is. While this state exists, it is difficult for me to make arrangements to live the rest of my days as a house-bound disabled person, because I do not believe that I should be in this position at all; I want help to get better, rather than help to maintain me in my illness. Unfortunately, this is the last thing the NHS is ever going to understand, or do something about.

So, I was kind of hoping that it would be xxxxxxx who 'told me' what I was going to need once at home. I can imagine a few basics; my ability to do anything at all at the moment is dependent on communication, for which I will need a good internet connection with a large, or preferably unlimited data plan. Once that is in place, most of my 'living' will be done online. Though I have always enjoyed cooking, utilising whatever foodstuffs came to hand, and using a wide range thereof, I now find myself in a position where it is distressing even to try this; I have diminishing strength and feeling and control in my hands and fingers, and have trouble focusing my eyes on what is in my hands and in my brain interpreting what my eyes are seeing. Thus I feel that I will have to be content with doing something I have recoiled from all my life, and getting ready cooked foods, and microwavable foods, home-delivered from the supermarkets. Writing this, I see that, horror of horrors, I may need an electric tin opener (when up until recently I would scoff at both tins and electric 'labour saving' gadgets!) Even having stuff delivered, I will still be a bit concerned at the putting away that follows. Even when I was helping others with this, I actually found the repeated bending and straightening after a home-delivery was actually worse than going shopping itself and, thus, knowing what was in each bag and exactly where it was going to be put. On my own, I won't need so much stuff, so I may be overstating the problem, and a few bags can be gradually put away over time... this said, I am, again, making the assumption that my sight doesn't further deteriorate. I cannot imagine me being able to learn how to communicate without sight enough to use a keyboard: once this has gone, I will be a vegetable.

At the moment, what happens when I try to do almost any physical activity is that my throat and chest quickly choke up as if I'm having an asthma attack, and then I have the sensation of air starvation and pain under my breastbone for hours, and often days, afterwards. I tried to hoover the entrance carpet here on Thursday, was choking within the minute, and my chest still aches and feels wheezy as I write. However, my reaction to this is not to want someone to do the sweeping etc. for me, but to want to get someone to force the NHS to find out why this happens, and fix it, so that I can get on and do stuff for myself! That is why it is difficult for me to contemplate what are my 'needs', let alone ask for help with them: my 'needs' have been artificially created by NHS negligence: the throat/ chest infection that is causing this choking breathlessness could be wiped out with a simple course of the right antibiotic, but I cannot even get doctors to try that simple measure! The very expression of my wish to get better confirms me in their eyes as a hypochondriac, so I simply cannot win.

Another thing that I expect I will have serious trouble with almost as soon as I am discharged is with the Department of Work and Pensions and Atos. Once I am not in 'hospital', I will become prey to the vultures at the DWP, who will try to deprive me of benefits and claim that I am now fit to work. As I cannot expect any help from my GP, who clearly does not believe what I am telling her of my symptoms, and, as my credibility has been destroyed by the libellous 'diagnosis' of 'hypochondriasis', I am going to need a very good advocate with experience in helping people with ME and other 'invisible' conditions get what they need to survive, with the minimum of harassment. However much as others may believe I'm only putting on some decades-long act, I cannot 'snap out of it'; do need benefits, and will die without them - unless the NHS can be persuaded to fix me, of course (which would surely be much cheaper in the long run!).

I can't even begin to explain to you how excruciating it is for me to watch other people doing my stuff for me. Doing everything for myself, my way, 'was' pretty much the whole of my life. If someone else is 'helping' by doing all this for me whilst I can only watch, I am in purgatory. Having to accept this, when I know that a competent diagnostician could probably identify and ameliorate the problem, is total hell.

I'm not sure I've helped you much by telling you all this. I have to rely on your good experience to try and put me right, as to the real needs of this stranger to himself!

Steve.

Dear World,

The life of ME:

This is the life of ME
From the person I was
To who this illness has made me be

Aching all over from head to toe
Moving clumsily
And walking so slow

This is the life of ME

Stomach swirling with a nauseous feeling
Certain foods are now less appealing

Head is pounding with pains and brain fogs
Longing to go for a walk with the dogs

This is the life of ME

Feeling drained twenty-four hours a day
Wishing this illness would go away

Trying to be normal, a mask on my face
Wondering how I got to this place

This is the life of ME

Lucky to have a network of support
Helping me through each battle I've fought

Who knows what else sufferers will have to endure
As we desperately wait and hope for a cure

By Emma xx

To those who don't knock before entering!

> ME and dignity...

There is a symptom of ME that shows up on no test, that has no tablet to relieve it, no cream to rub on.

Is it pain I speak of, or fatigue, or malaise? Maybe the motion sickness, light sensitivity, brain fog? No, none of those, although for sure they are there.

I talk of dignity, or lack of. The complete loss of personal space, of independence. The rape of private life.

Invasion by carers. Seeing you daily whether you like it or not. Letting themselves in with a key that hangs outside. Having someone wash you, feed you. Unwanted intimacy. In and out of your bedroom when they choose despite the 'Do Not Disturb' sign which hangs there. Managing your home the way they like, touching your stuff, the rooms you have no access to. As if they know best.

'They're just doing their job', you say, 'life would be impossible without them'. This I well know. That makes it worse.

And dare I mention the commode? Not being able to stand to shut the curtains as double-deckers go by? No, I won't go there, that's for your imagination.

Friends complain that I refuse their visits. 'Can't they just pop their head round the door and say hi?' Apart from the symptoms this would cause me, the energy consumption used, meaning I have to forgo my precious forty minutes of telly, or washing my feet, or a phone call to my mum... aside from that, I really don't want to be seen. At my worst. At my most vulnerable. Feeling like death, looking like a corpse.

Funny how people feel they can comment on my appearance. 'Your skin's looking bad. You've put on weight. You're looking thinner', as if I didn't know. Believe me, I feel how I look. I know. Thanks.

I rarely look in the mirror, but what do I see when I do? Blanched, grey skin, too long without sunlight. That unmistakable green ME tinge around the eyes. Hair lank, dirty, peculiar chunks where I cut bits off. An expression screaming disease and fatigue, disgust at its reflection.

'But you're ill, these things don't matter, it's the least of your problems'. I know that too, yet shame still remains.

My wardrobe full of outfits I cannot wear. Of beautiful shoes and handbags. Jewellery, those vain baubles, meaningless yet so meaningful. How I long to colour co-ordinate, to wear clothes instead of nightwear, pretty undies instead of comfort.

'Vanity equals sanity' I had someone say. So I paint my nails, I sigh, and I dream of vibrance, of beauty, of what I hope to be again, if age doesn't overtake me whilst I wait here for health.

From me... xx

To everyone around me,

Why do people ask what made me decide to up working, even though I had reduced my week to only fifteen hours? This of course often became twenty-five hours in order for me to get the work done, now that I am struggling so much.

I started to dread going down the stairs at work because that meant that I would have to go up them again. I was finding it extremely difficult to sustain an interest in clients during meetings. I had also begun to lose my voice again when having a conversation that lasted longer than ten minutes, so coping with one-hour appointments or lengthy training sessions was becoming an impossibility.

People started to comment about how ill I looked, and I was experiencing chest pains and breathing difficulties that came on in the same way as when I first had the chronic fatigue.

Occasionally my arm ached so much after a phone call that I could not move it to put the phone down. I found myself forgetting words as I spoke and often had to stop half-way through a word because I could not end it. Often the word I wanted to say would come out backwards, or I would say the complete opposite of the word I was planning to say.

I was losing out on any kind of a life outside of work. This was because I needed more and more rest to cope with my few half-days working. Everything had become too much of an effort. If I had visitors at home, I would need to plan three or four hours rest before they came and then make sure I went straight to bed after they left.

I feel my husband's patience is wearing thin now, because he is used to me doing so much for the home and our business in the past. I have decided to give some charity notes to family members for them to read.

I dream about the days when I could:

Do the housework
Go shopping, do cooking, washing etc.
Go to keep fit
Swim
Play squash
Walk the dog
Have a full-time job
...and socialise.

From Kelly.

Dear judgemental people,

You stare at me, you look and think, 'is she faking', or am I a missing link?

As I pull up into the blue badge space, I couldn't look any more out of place.

People stare, they watch and snigger, does that really make you feel any bigger?

Would you like me to crawl out of the car? Would you like my appearance to look strange and bizarre?

No I'm not elderly, my body looks fine, I haven't lost a leg, or broken my spine.

But out of the boot, my wheelchair comes, whilst people are sat there, twiddling their thumbs.

'Does she need that?', 'is there anything wrong?', 'this blue badge space is not where she belongs!'

Why is this? Because I'm young and look healthy? Do you deserve this space more, because you're old and wealthy?

What do you have to judge a girl like me? What is it that you need to see?

My wheelchair comes round, right up to my door. But that's not enough, they want some more.

I wish I could see through my brave face, I wish you could see the pain I have to embrace.

What you need to know, is my illness hides, not every disability can be seen from the outside.

So next time you see me pull into that space, don't bother staring, put a smile on your face.

I may not look ill, but I'm fighting and strong. This blue badge space is where, at the moment, I do belong.

Lots of love, Kate x

Hello, yes, I'm talking to you.

I saw you staring; you didn't even try to hide it. I saw the confusion on your face when you heard me speak, when you saw me take a few steps. I saw the disbelief when I held an intelligent conversation with a friend, when I purchased my shopping by myself.

I saw the horror in your eyes when I asked you to help me reach something, or open a door. Do you think being in a wheelchair is catching? Or maybe you assume I must be mentally disabled too.

Believe it or not I am bright, I study, I drive, I sew, I read and my wheelchair has no connection to my brain.

My health has taken a lot of opportunities away from me but I am still a human being. I'm still here, I'm still the person I was five years ago before I got sick.

Look past the wheelchair and see the person inside it, we're in 2014 not 1914 - there is nothing to fear.

From Hannah xxx

To all the people who have made my physical illness more distressing and damaging than it should have and could have been,

To the psychiatrist who shouted at me and told me I was lazy when I said I couldn't exercise every day because of my ME. Firstly, you are supposed to treat all patients with care and respect, not make value judgements and humiliate them. Secondly, you were supposed to be treating my depression and anxiety; whilst I am aware that exercise is helpful to people with depression, your refusal to then discuss my mental health or medication changes shows that YOU are a LAZY doctor. Why tax your brain to try to help someone when you can just shout at them and send them away?

To the next psychiatrist who referred to my ME as 'motivation disorder' in a referral letter. If you have diagnosed me with this disorder, why were you not attempting to treat it? More to the point, how can you say that someone to whom you repeatedly turned down requests to go on depression counselling waiting lists is unmotivated? Does someone who is unmotivated repeatedly engage in attempts to improve her mental and physical health, and her situation, and cause repeated relapses with attempts to complete a degree course?

To all the GPs and psychiatrists who didn't believe or care that I had severe insomnia. I am no longer sleep deprived thanks to a doctor who believed and medicated me. I'm still physically ill, but now that I get adequate, restful sleep I may be able to work part-time and visit my friends, and just live a little more. You could have made that difference years ago but you were too arrogant and too dismissive.

To the people with ME that I knew before I was ill or diagnosed, and your spiteful 'congratulations' and 'you've got what you wanted' when I reached out to you after my diagnosis. You'd found me guilty of being 'one of those people who wants to say they have ME for sympathy' because of a simple mix up on my part between CFS and post-viral fatigue. I most certainly didn't want ME; at the time I wanted an explanation for my excessive tiredness, weakness and constantly feeling ill. I'd only ever been kind and tried to help you both. You not only denied me any kindness, but your attitude towards me made me shy away from contact with other people with ME. I was completely isolated for years; I didn't get any of the positive support and valuable information from fellow sufferers. Did I really deserve that?

To the other people with ME that have implied or said that I don't have ME because I have already suffered from depression, and because my health has improved due to anti-depressants. You KNOW what it's like to have your physical illness dismissed as psychosomatic - why would you inflict that on someone else? My glands have been swollen to the size of golf balls for the entire length of my illness; I don't know of any psychiatric disorder that is a symptom of! The anti-depressants treat my insomnia, I get more sleep, I have better health - it's not rocket science.

For those people who knew me as a child and teenager. I didn't like PE and sports and was kind of lazy because I was slow and rubbish at those things. I was a complete drama queen and hypochondriac and used to get out of doing things by saying I was ill. I am NOT that child now. I grew up, I worked very hard in an extremely stressful job for a few years, and I only went off on long-term sick leave when Occupational Health recommended it. I left and I worked hard to make it through the first year of a degree that I loved, despite being more and more ill. I continued doing my daily cardio workout and pushed on with the second year of my degree, even after I was diagnosed and advised to stop both. I literally pushed myself to the point of collapse.

Finally to those people who say 'we all get tired', or some other such dismissive statements. How often are you so exhausted you have to lie down simply because you had a shower and got dressed? How often do you feel so weak that you can't stand long enough for the kettle to boil and then you can't even lift the kettle to pour it? How often do you have to ask your partner to help you out of bed to use the toilet because you don't have the strength to get there quickly enough on your own? I'm not just tired; I'm often exhausted by very small activity. I feel ill ALL the time. My good days are how you feel when you've got a heavy cold and not had enough sleep, my bad days are like the flu; my body is made of lead and the duvet feels like sandbags crushing me. I'm in pain all the time; sometimes just a dull ache in joints and limbs, sometimes a throbbing fire or sharp lightning. I'm not going to list the myriad of other symptoms, but every single part of my body is affected, even my intelligence and memory; sometimes I can't even remember my own date of birth. I have to monitor my symptoms, not because I'm a hypochondriac but I need to try to prevent myself from crashing into a relapse, or from missing signs of things that might need medical intervention. Still, it's very unpredictable and variable.

I know it's hard to really understand someone's life unless you live it, but anyone who really knows me will know that I'd give my right arm to be working, exercising, seeing the world, making a difference if I had the choice. I am one of the lucky ones, because I can have those good days, I can go out and have snippets of a normal life, but sadly they come at a cost and it means I can't have them all the time; I can't hold down a job and can't live completely independently. Some can't even leave their beds or their homes, have you ever been that tired? For weeks, months, years on end?

From C.

This is for all you people out there who make our lives a nightmare, yeah

Don't say nuthin' if it ain't worth, don't say nuthin' if it ain't worth worth worth, don't say nuthin' if it ain't worth, don't say nuthin' if it ain't worthwhile.

**********X*******

It's like a magnet under the ground pulling ya down till ya on ya knees

Fighting this disease, can't breathe, muscles cease, pain is a pain that you would not believe

And you have the audacity to say I look fine, whatever's going on is going on in my mind

Yeah well come tell me that when I'm flat, laying on my back like a knick knack paddy whack no energy yeah, come see, then ya pray ya never get ME

**********X*********

It's like treacle ya trying to run, ya head says go but ya body's saying uh uh

I ain't doing that, but I don't wanna wheelchair, my mama's my carer she got a lot to bear

I get frustrated angry and cross, I shout at the main man for the life that I've lost

But that's OK, it's just a bad day, we're all entitled to feel that way

But if I get out I put on a face, walking happy and confident, you won't see a trace

Just coz you don't see it, don't mean it ain't there, to judge us on that is totally unfair

Come do that when I'm flat, laying on my back like a knick knack, paddy whack, struggling with disability yeah, come see, then ya pray ya never get ME

**********X**********

Don't say nuthin' if it ain't worth, (shuuuuuuutuuuuup) don't say nuthin' if it ain't worth worth worth, don't say nuthin' if it ain't worth, don't say nuthin' if it ain't worthwhile.

Don't say nuthin' if it ain't worth, (shuuuuuuutuuuuup) don't say nuthin' if it ain't worth worth worth, don't say nuthin' if it ain't worth, don't say nuthin' if it ain't worthwhile

**********X**********

It's like being drunk, ya trying to talk, ya words get slurred and ya stagger when ya walk

Memory's bad, it happens a lot, go to say something an'............................I forgot

It's really kinda weird like a brain malfunction, there's people out there who've come to the assumption, we're making it up, putting it on, needing attention and that's why it's done

Yeah well come tell me that when I'm flat, laying on my back like a knick knack paddy whack,

& It's hurting to breathe, yeah come see, then ya pray ya never get ME

***********X**********

It's like waking up every day feeling as though ya dying

Tha worlds hating on ya & theres no way of replying

To tha media attacks from tha hacks that haven't got a clue

creating hullabaloo

Nuthin's ever changing, ignorance is rife

It's just words to you, but its... our... life... life... life... life

*************x***********

It's like half a dozen people sitting on ya shoulder, aching all over, gonna throw up

Heads all dizzy, insides fizzy, knock, knock, knock, but the doors are shut

No concentration, all spaced out, welcome to ME and what some of it's about,

And if you don't believe that when I'm flat laying on my back like a knick knack paddy whack,

No energy, coping with disability, & it's hurting to breathe, and you still can't see? Just pray ya never get ME

*************x***********

Don't say nuthin' if it ain't worth, (shuuuuuuutuuuuup) don't say nuthin' if it ain't worth worth worth, don't say nuthin' if it ain't worth, don't say nuthin' if it ain't worthwhile.

Don't say nuthin' if it ain't worth, don't say nuthin' if it ain't worth worth worth, don't say nuthin' if it ain't worth, don't say nuthin' if it ain't worthwhile

© Mama Chill

To anyone who thinks they know what I'm going through,

I've seen how you look at me. You think you know everything, and I can almost see the words blasting out from you, the whole 'there's nothing wrong with you', the whole 'you're making this up', the whole 'you want attention' thing.

You presume that because I don't look ill in front of you, this is all a lie. That is where you are wrong. Know this before you judge me.

When I'm not with you, I often lie screaming in pain. Sometimes I would rather die than have to tolerate the feeling of being crushed, or burnt, or ripped apart. Sometimes the pain is so severe I am unable to do anything, but merely cry. When you have felt such pain, then you can judge me.

When I'm not with you, my brain is so foggy I can't put a sentence together. Sometimes, I can't remember who people are, even my friends and family. Sometimes, I have to witness and feel awful at the faces of those people, the hurt and embarrassment that I don't know them - the embarrassment that I feel. When you have felt such humiliation, then you can judge me.

When I'm not with you, I experience really awful sensitivities. Sometimes, I can't cope with a hug from a friend because it hurts me so much, even though that's all I want in the world. Sometimes, someone opening my bedroom door makes my head pound - I'm so sensitive to the noise that it is like a huge thunder clap in my ear. Sometimes, I ask if we can go and eat somewhere with more choice because I can't tolerate gluten (the times that I have risked it, I have made myself extremely ill). When you have felt so ill from such small triggers, then you can judge me.

When I'm not with you, it is a massive achievement for me to walk around my house. Sometimes, it feels like climbing the stairs is climbing Kilimanjaro. Sometimes, I have to use plastic cutlery because metal is too heavy. Sometimes, it feels like a marathon just to even walk into the bathroom to clean my teeth and back to my bedroom. When you have felt so drained after doing such small activities, then you can judge me.

I try to keep my suffering to a minimum when I'm with you, because you judge me enough. You see me every day and I look fine - and you judge me enough from that alone. I can't face the thought of you picking away at the real suffering that goes on behind closed doors. You rarely say anything to me to my face, but I know you talk when I'm not there. Just because I have an illness it doesn't make me stupid. But know that those odd comments deeply hurt me. The odd 'OH MY GOD - I can't listen to you go on about that again'. The odd 'oh right... but you look fine'. That makes me feel completely useless. Literally useless. As though the fight that I go through every day to appear as normal as possible to you is worth nothing, and that makes me feel like nothing. But I always try to forgive you, to tell myself that you've never been in my shoes so you can't possibly understand. All I need now is for you to see that there is so much you don't see. So much that you don't feel. I hope you never will.

When you have had ME, then you can judge me.

Victoria xxxxxx

To everyone who has doubted the severity...

>A moment of severe ME.

Imagine the worst flu you've ever had. The pain in muscles and joints, the fever, the miserable malaise and weakness. Then add to that the worst hangover you have known. The nausea, vomiting and retching, the dizziness and sickening headache, the feeling that you've been poisoned.

Stir in the disrupted sleep pattern and exhaustion of jet-lag, the confused mental sluggishness. Now double it, triple it, and you are somewhat close to what it feels like to have ME.

Sound, like fireworks going off in your mind, sending blasts of light through your brain, shockwaves of searing pain through your body. Movement, causing the room to spin, your stomach to leap, your body to rock.

Burning eyes and skin, like you are packed in dry ice, tingling and buzzing in every fibre. Teeth chattering and limbs shaking at every minor task. Your body rejecting food, light, smells... everything that makes up a day.

'But it's called Chronic Fatigue Syndrome' I hear you say. Ah yes, the fatigue. The feeling like you've been bled. Like your bones have been replaced with lead pipes, your muscles with sandbags. The fatigue so great that you are unable to move, speak, open your eyes. Unsure whether you can draw another breath.

'Surely it can't be that bad, surely you can't feel that ill, not for so long?' Years, my friend. And there enters the hopelessness, the despair, the terror of the next moment. The disbelief that you can feel so unbearably ill and yet not die.

The longing for independence, for dignity. The yearning to escape the coffin sized space you are confined to, to feel the wind on your skin, to see birds and grass again. To be with family you are unable to allow near you, any friends you have left. Even a casual stroll round a supermarket would be an ultimate highlight.

So please, don't tell me I'm enjoying the attention, the lack of responsibility, being waited upon. Don't say I'm not trying hard enough; I'm obsessed with self and consumed by my health.

Am I paranoid about catching viruses and infections? I ask you, would you want to feel any worse than this?

Every day I climb a mountain in physical effort, take a degree in mental output, and win gold in sheer determination and grit. Please do congratulate me for the strength I show in this day. For by doing so, you will help me get through another.

Xxxxx

To those who refuse to believe in ME,
> Disbelief at the disbelief.

I'm not ill, you say? I am imagining my symptoms? Making this up? I am honestly dumbfounded at what you come out with.

I'm afraid of getting well? Don't want the responsibility? I enjoy the attention? Whose attention do you think I'm getting? I see no-one.

I choose this life? I'm happy to live like this? I don't want to recover? So would you accept a life of isolation, pain, stillness? Darkness, weakness, unimaginable fatigue? An illness with over a hundred symptoms listed. One compared with an AIDs sufferer a few weeks from death, of someone undergoing chemotherapy...

An estimated seventeen million sufferers worldwide. More prevalent than lung cancer, leukemia and AIDS combined. We can't ALL be making his up, can't ALL be imagining it, surely? And why would we for goodness sake?

Disbelief from doctors, disbelief from family, disbelief from friends... then comes the criticism - I do nothing to help myself, I refuse treatment, I exaggerate... then comes the suggestions - I need to get outdoors, a good steak, a long walk, anti-depressants, this therapy... that therapy...

Then follows fear. Fear of what the doctors will do to me, fear of being forced into hospital. Threats of psychiatric wards, Cognitive Behaviour Therapy, Graded Exercise Therapy... knowing the devastating effect this would have, yet being unable to convince. How can I get them to understand? Do I beg?

I wish what you say were true, that this is all in my mind, that I can think myself well, mind over matter. I would then be healthy tomorrow! But no, I am in this bedridden state due to an unexplained medical condition.

It cannot be understood therefore it cannot exist? Yet I exist.

An ME sufferer.

To anyone who doesn't believe that ME is a real physical disease,

Well, you are entitled to your beliefs. However, you need to realise that in this case your beliefs contradict over fifty years' of scientific research, the World Health Organisation, and the experiences of millions of patients around the world.

On what grounds do you not believe in it? If it's because it's invisible, well, do you also disbelieve those with broken legs? Or cancer? Or diabetes?

Or is it because the treatment recommendations - to rest and to be careful to not do things that cause an increase in symptoms - are so different to the recommendations given for other diseases? I can understand it seeming counterintuitive and being hard to get your head around – but that doesn't mean it's not true (the research is out there if you want to read it!) or that it isn't vital for ME sufferers to follow those recommendations.

Is it because you just can't believe that so many people's lives could be so severely affected, and yet the medical profession has nothing constructive to offer them? (Believe me, we sufferers find this one hard to get our heads round, too.)

I'm pretty sure it's at least partly because you've never known anyone with ME – or not known them closely, anyway. You may have seen so-called mild or moderate sufferers on their good days, the days when they've rested beforehand and so are able to keep their 'brave face' mask on for a few hours – but you haven't seen the awful payback that they have to go through afterwards, and you haven't seen the sacrifices they have to make just to grab those few hours of pretending to be normal. And you've not seen the desperate struggles that severe sufferers go through daily, just to keep going. You've not seen the severe physical agony. You've not seen the dozens of bizarre neurological, endocrine, and immunological symptoms ('fatigue' is such a misnomer; ME is far, far more than that, and ME sufferers would give anything to be 'just' fatigued). You've not seen the frustration when they want to talk or eat, but their facial muscles won't work so they have to wait until their muscles co-operate again. You've not seen the huge effort they put into just taking a few steps on a good day. You've not seen the indignity they have to endure, of having strangers in their home, strangers giving them a wash or feeding them. And you've not seen their joy in small achievements or their delightfully dark humour; you've not seen their fighting spirit or their hope that, one day, things might be a bit better. Maybe you think they're just lazy, or maybe you think they're agoraphobic or just depressed – but ME doesn't take away our ability to see beauty in the world, to yearn for the outside world.

I read somewhere that one way to tell the difference between someone who is depressed and someone who has ME without depression is to ask them what they'd do if they got well. A person with depression will probably say something along the lines of 'don't know'. They won't be able to imagine feeling OK again, they won't feel an interest in life, they won't see the potential for beauty or fun or excitement in life. A person with ME, however, will probably give you a long list of things they want to do, things they're excited about, things they hope for.

No-one in their right mind would believe that they were this sick if it wasn't really true, if they could help it. The darkest imagination could not dream up this level of devastating suffering. I hope you and your loved ones never get ME – but, if you did, if you truly experienced the reality of ME, your views on it would change very very quickly.

There is more and more research proving damage and dysfunction in various systems in ME sufferers' bodies, and more and more research is backing up what ME sufferers have been saying all along. So don't tell me that this disease isn't real. If you must persist in believing that, against all the evidence, then that's your choice – but keep your outdated and ignorant beliefs to yourself. Don't tell me that I'm scared to go out, don't tell me that I should be trying a bit harder – it's a huge slap in the face when actually I'm desperate to experience the outside world again, I long to feel the wind on my face again, I yearn to run and swim and hike and hundreds of other activities. I love life, I enjoy life, and I want to experience it to the full – but I can't, because this stupid disease makes my body unco-operative, and because ME isn't a 'cool' disease so doesn't attract much research funding. But I'll keep hoping and fighting and supporting those who are working towards a cure. While I'm waiting for a cure, I'll keep fighting and doing all I can to maximise my health. And if a cure comes within my lifetime, well, look out world! There's so much I want to do and experience – I hope you're ready for me!

Xx

Dear Me...

A letter to myself before ME, my healthy self,

Please take care of yourself and do not take your health for granted. Slow down and appreciate what you have; enjoy every walk, rambling through the hills, stop and enjoy the scenery and take deep breaths of that beautiful air, listen to the waterfalls, appreciate the flowers and birds - for it will not always be so.

Appreciate every family gathering, listen to the chatter of your extended family, eat, drink, laugh, dance and take time to notice what is happening - for it will not always be so.

Enjoy your holidays skiing as fast as you can, run along beaches, try all the fastest rides at Disneyland, learn to water-ski and do that bungee jump, slow down and appreciate every moment - for it will not always be so.

Enjoy your work but do not push yourself too hard, when you feel tired rest, when you are unwell take time off, appreciate what you are good at and realise that you are successful and you do not need to keep doing more and more, slow down and appreciate what you have achieved - for it will not always be so.

Enjoy your healthy body full of vitality; run, ride, swim, dance, sing, jump, act, climb trees but slow down and appreciate what you can do. Don't expect too much from yourself, look after that vibrant shell - for it will not always be so.

Enjoy your inquisitive mind, read a range of books, talk and discuss things that interest you, do puzzles, discuss mathematical problems, write articles, investigate problems, recite poetry and learn languages but take time to appreciate what you can do - for it will not always be so.

From your future me x

Message to myself twelve years ago,

If I could use the time portal as in Star Trek I would go back in time and tell myself about this illness. These are the things I would say:

- Take it seriously from day one

- Don't push yourself

- Don't do Graded Exercise

- Change your doctor earlier to one more sympathetic and understanding

- Don't resign from your job but push for ill health retirement

- Don't force yourself to work at any cost

- Don't take on a new job when you know deep down that you are not well

- Be honest with yourself about your abilities and your health

- Find out more about the illness

- Realise that it's not going away and will be with you for the rest of your life

- Accept it sooner and not fight against it

- Know that you will have some bad and good periods

- Avoid stress as much as possible as it will only make you worse

- Don't assume that you will get better

- Plan your life according to the restrictions of the illness

- Relax more

- Don't waste time trying to convince family and friends that you are truly ill

- Rest and pace as much as possible

- Say 'no' more often

- Don't be bullied into doing things that are too much for you

- Don't worry about the jobs you can't do and take better care of yourself

- Push for more help and support from the medical profession

- And above all know that life will go on, albeit not the same

I wonder if I'd had all that help and advice, would things have been different?

Me, in the future x

To my future healthy self,

I am writing to you now, hoping against hope that you are real, that in my future there is a healthy self waiting for me - a self who has long since recovered from ME. If you are real, if I am headed on a journey towards a healthy future, then I have some things I'd like to ask that you do.

Take joy in every day. Every time you wake up and don't feel extreme pain, take joy. Every time you walk around without it being painful or exhausting, take joy. Never forget the pain you once felt, so that you can take joy in its absence.

Remember how lucky you are to have good health, and enjoy it. Enjoy your life. Do things you enjoy, spend quality time with your friends and family, laugh every day. Give freely to others, now that you have the health to do so. Follow all of your dreams, now that your health isn't holding you back.

I don't know how long the novelty lasted once you regained your health, but I really hope you didn't get bogged down by your daily routine and stop being thankful every day for your recovery, and forget to be eternally grateful. If so, stop for a moment and re-connect with your feelings on losing your diagnosis and realising you had recovered. Don't ever let those feelings stray too far.

I hope that you appreciate it all the time and are happy living a life free of ME. I know life can throw lots of hard times your way in manners unrelated to health, but if you have a really rough day remember the pain and the exhaustion you once suffered every day, remember you now have the health and energy to tackle your problems; contemplate how much worse your situation would be with severely ill health added on top.

Please don't forget all of your friends left behind who still have ME - be there for them and support them with their journey as they supported you with yours. They are truly amazing people, who brightened up the life of your past self, so please make sure to save time for them.

Raise your children to also take joy in every day, to laugh often, to appreciate their health, their family and friends, and to find happiness in the simple things.

And finally, if you exist, please be always thankful, because at this point it looks doubtful that you, my healthy self, will ever come into being. If by a miracle you do, please do not waste the opportunity. Be true to yourself and follow some of the many hopes and dreams I currently have for you or any others that develop over time.

May the rest of your life be happy and healthy.

Your former self

Dear ME,

I have tried to summarise you in my piece below, but nothing I could ever write would adequately describe the loss, pain and heartache as well as the disability and symptoms that you have brought to me, but also to my family over the years. For that I can never forgive you, especially as you continue to bring so much misery to me and to all of the other lovely, caring people I know who also battle each day with a vast variety of disabling symptoms. They are so misunderstood, and in some cases sadly not even believed.

You have taken so much from so many, ME. From the things people used to enjoy and love right down to their very independence. This is indeed true for me. This letter is for all of those who doubted me, disbelieved me and for all of the countless acts of ignorance and unkindness I have endured over the years.

You came into my life ME, suddenly and without warning after a nasty virus that left me reeling with nausea and vomiting. I returned to school for a short while but the virus-like state never went away, in fact it just got worse. I struggled through the remainder of the term feeling nauseous, dizzy and weak and was completely shattered by the afternoons, coming home only to stagger up to bed. I didn't have the energy to complete homework nor to take part in activities I enjoyed.

What was happening to me? My local GP was unable to give me an answer, but one doctor mentioned that I was more than likely to be suffering from post-viral fatigue syndrome and I would be better in a few months. Even sitting on my pony now became too much of a task, leaving me feeling sick and exhausted.

Getting into school was even more challenging. I wanted to keep pushing myself, I wanted to study and I wanted to play sports but each time I tried the illness just seemed to get worse. It just didn't seem fair.

I spent countless lessons in pain and considerable sickness, but each time I approached the school nurse I was just sent back into class. I was made to feel inadequate and disbelieved. I could see my education, confidence and everything around me falling apart before my eyes.

As my health declined so my battles with doctors grew. I was made to feel as if it were all my fault; that I wasn't trying hard enough and, ultimately, as if I were somehow responsible or exaggerating my symptoms. Doctors used to tell me that it was clear that I just didn't want to go to school and that I would never achieve anything if I kept up this game. Their attacks and also their manner upset me greatly and I would leave consultations crying and shaking rigid that professionals could be so threatening and unkind. No-one who turns to the health system for help should be made to feel that way. No matter what the circumstance.

It felt as though we as a family seemed to be being swept up in a tornado storm, battered and bashed and battered some more with no remorse. We were just drifting further and further away from help.

Thankfully I registered with a new doctor and I am now building up strong trust. He is kind, concerned and approachable, taking the lead from me from the very first day that we met. Finally, two years on from first developing symptoms I was referred to a specialist service who deals with ME/ Chronic Fatigue Syndrome. The consultant diagnosed me almost immediately with moderate to severe ME. At long last I knew what was wrong but by now my education and life were in tatters.

Trips to the hospital remain just as challenging. I still feel as if I am being looked upon in a different light from other patients. My symptoms remain a constant, ever-changing battle and I struggle to deal with the disability. They are vast, unrelenting and exhausting and affect most, if not all, of my body systems. I now have to use a wheelchair. I am in too much pain; too exhausted and unbalanced. I still have many challenges and uncertainties ahead of me. Not the least is where, ME, you have left my education and my future.

One thing I do know is that this planet will always spin on, oblivious to the struggles of those who rattle around on its surface. Very few people will stop and wait for you. I now know what it feels like to become shut out, isolated and forgotten. To feel stranded and helpless. To become lost in a separate world of seemingly endless physical suffering.

I do feel as though it is time that we didn't have to feel so alone. Time that we felt as though we had solid support in all areas of educational, pastoral and medical care. For professionals to become more aware of all of the multiple and complex symptoms that can arise, so people will be able to receive the appropriate diagnosis within the first three to six months of developing illness. The delay in diagnosis and lack of understanding only prolongs and increases the severity of the disability and the chances of full recovery. I feel as though we should not have to endure such ignorance and unkindness for something that just isn't our fault. All we ask for is to be believed and for our care to be appropriately managed. Maybe then fewer lives will be turned completely upside down like mine has.

For all of your support Mum, I will always be so grateful.

Holly Buckley, 16.

My stomach always queasy with legs uneasy
The room lurching and my head swirling
Every part of my body burning
With constant, unrelenting pain.

My eyes now feel heavy
and I'm always unsteady.
Sometimes I feel so weak
I forget what I'm saying when I speak.

Each drop of energy just seems to drains away
Leaving me shattered, unable to think, lifeless and pale.

I'm sixteen and stuck behind the same four walls
For most of the day
All opportunities and everything I once loved
Now cruelly taken away.

My life passes me by in a hazy blur
Each day feels the same but some even worse
It just doesn't seem fair
When it feels like there is no-one to turn to
And no-one is there.

Disbelief and doubts just add to the pain
I couldn't even begin to explain
How it feels to feel this way
And then to be given the blame

What would it be like to feel normal again?
To enjoy life without payback, symptoms and pain
To ride a bike or take a stroll
Even if the clouds were grey
I long to be free for just one day.

What saddens me most
Is that few people really know
What you, ME, are like and why you never go
How awful you make me feel every single day,
You are a long, lonely nightmare that just won't go away.

Dear ME Diagnosis,

You come of age this month! September 1995 and still there. I'd rather you went away, but I guess that is rather too much to ask.

I managed to thwart you for a bit and go back to part-time work for a couple of years... but I could often feel your shadow stealing back over me, only too eager to claim me as your own.

You were lying in wait and when I wasn't looking you hit me with a nasty bout of your favourite 'flu - you put me back into bed and truly back into your evil clutches.

Currently you give me more bad days than good. But the worst thing is you're letting me make plans that never get fulfilled.

One day I would love to wake up and not feel exhausted... but you remind me within seconds of waking that you are still there!

One day I would love to be out of my bed all day and being busy like I used to... but you are always lurking just round the corner with your 'Post Exertional Malaise', wild temperatures and hatred of noise, light and smells!

If anyone mentions one more time that 'pacing' might help beat you then I will scream. But that would only be wasted energy.

And, as if that's not enough, you force me to do battle with the Department of Work and Pension's longest and silliest forms as you've robbed me of my ability to work more than a couple of hours a week.

But I am still here.

I would cheerfully celebrate your passing... but suspect your tenacity will help you survive well into adulthood.

But I still survive as me.

I have friends who have put up with me longer than you've

been around and know you all too well, and others who still struggle to understand your callous nature.

So you see, ME, you will not win!

You cannot stop me being me, even though you want YOU to be more important.

I am me first and ME second.

Please remember that!

Jane

A rant to ME;

I'm furious with you for coming into my daughter's life! She is so sick she can no longer get out of bed; she is having visual, olfactory and auditory hallucinations, intermittent paralysis of her legs, and has nausea so badly that she can only eat over-cooked, plain, boiled pasta or rice along with sips of water. When she does eat the food just goes straight through her and leaves her exhausted, clammy and scared.

Why have you done this to her? What has this poor child done to deserve this? She is only fifteen years old - you arrived almost two years ago and you have robbed her of her childhood, her ability to have an education, party, be with friends. You have stripped away her confidence, her ambition, her laughter. She thinks she is dying - she doesn't believe an illness like ME can make you feel so awful for so long. She sees her sister, who has had ME for almost four years STILL suffering badly too - and wonders if anyone EVER improves or gets stronger from being this ill.

She now thinks that the doctors have got it wrong and that she MUST have terminal cancer - she feels so ill that every minute of every day is a struggle. I just wish there was something I could do to help make her feel better, to bring back the laughter and the hope - to see the light back in her eyes. Her sister is a little more hopeful, but then she was never as sick as this. I want answers, I want help, I want understanding from the public - not snipes of how I am enabling the girls to 'believe' they are sick - that they just need to be pushed to get out of bed and get on with life! Most of all I WANT treatments to help improve their quality of life.

Signed by a frustrated, devastated and heartbroken mother.

Dear ME,

You came into my life at a vital age, when I was supposed to be doing GCSE's and dancing every day. Fourteen is so young to have your life tipped around and be so scared about the future. It started with tiredness, and then came the pain; I lost so much weight that I was days from getting hospitalised and tube-fed. Doctors had no clue and told me it was depression and anorexia, but why couldn't you see that I was so anxious because I didn't know what was the matter? Four-hour panic attacks every day for months, and I had so little energy I started crawling up the stairs and got stuck in bed. A year later I got my diagnosis, but no advice. No help, no medicine, just 'you'll be better by summer'.

I left confused. I left feeling alone. What was I supposed to do now? An officer came to our house and told my mum she'd go to jail if I didn't go to school the next day, so several panic attacks later I forced myself in. I remember my friend coming to hug me after months of not seeing me. She wrapped her arms around me, then recoiled saying 'oh my God'. By this point every bone was sticking out of me. My legs were just bone and my waist got so small. So rumours started, Kate won't eat. False. Kate can't eat. You don't understand.

School were useless. Not moving classrooms downstairs when I couldn't walk. Only providing four weeks of fifteen minute lessons of home schooling a day to do my WHOLE GCSEs. Their view was I was clever so I'd be OK. It was OK to forget about me. After a struggle with them I was told to take a year out, breaking my heart as school was the thing that kept me focused. So I left.

The next year is a blur. I remember getting very poorly. I remember paralysis. I remember not being able to brush my own teeth or feed myself. I stared at my wall all day and that was it. I didn't give up though. I remember the first time I stood up for ten seconds with my physio holding me, my legs shaking uncontrollably but I was so happy. And from then on, I took more steps, little by little, and got myself to where I am today.

I started an online course. This eventually led to me starting part-time college. I learnt so much on my journey. I started volunteering and became a leader for my county. I started raising money and awareness for ME. I started to give my friends hope that I once lost, showing them my journey. I would never have known I had such a talent in textiles, or got the opportunity to teach ballet, or met so many friends. My friends keep me strong when times are tough. I've got a small circle of amazing friends who have ME who inspire me every day to keep going. And I hope I give that back to them.

So to all the doctors who told me it was in my head. All the physiotherapists who said I might not walk again. All my school friends who left me. Well, thank you. You made me the person I am today - 100% stronger and appreciative.

Kate Stanforth

To the vile, debilitating illness that has stolen three whole entire years (so far) of my teen life. Thanks a million; I won't get them back!

Do I dare ask why you feel the need to create such agony and heart-ache, fear and uncertainty in my life? Will you punish me even more?

Why on earth did you chose ME - what have I done to upset you? Why couldn't you choose somebody who doesn't want to do anything with their life - someone who doesn't want to create a journey of wisdom, or someone who doesn't want to live life to the full? I am not that somebody! I want to get good grades, I want to go out, enjoy myself and cherish countless numbers of memorable teenage moments, I want to travel; but most importantly, I want to dance!!

Due to the fact that you have chosen me, I have to live every day as it comes. I can't plan or do what I like when I like; instead I suffer with overwhelming, chronic pain, day after day - some days you push it further, you exhaust me, paralyse me, leaving me for hours in a situation I dread, leaving me in a surge of suspense. You have torn me away from the one thing I rely on to escape from the world for a little while. You have beaten me up, ripped out my soul and left me in a place I deeply loathe. I can't escape from this. You are harshly in control. You've tied me to an anchor, thrown me into deep waters and left me to drown...

My main ambition in life is to become a professional dancer - but I already know that you know that! You're torturing me - I can feel your evil within me.

You've crushed my dreams for so many years now. Why can't you let me go? I beg you to stop holding on to me - I want to be free!

I often hear that I will feel worse before I get better, but that's not the case for you! You decide to drag me onto a roller-coaster ride, making every relapse longer and stronger - giving me false hope when I feel so well!

I don't understand how millions of people believe that you're fake? You're so real to me! Doctors think I'm crazy, and that I need psychological help. I'm told that I'm 'imaging the pain' and that 'it's all in my head'. They're wrong. You know they are! You just like the entertainment of seeing me struggle. You feed from the insomnia, the dizziness, the nausea. You enjoy it when I scream and cry from the several types of pain and horrible sensations - you poke me like a voodoo doll.

I hate you.

However, I have a surprise for you! I would like to thank you! Thank you for making me strong-willed. Thank you for making me put up a fight! You are still hitting me hard, but nowadays the ever so small achievements make me feel so happy! I've pushed grades up from E's and F's to C's and B's, and I achieved an A* in my GCSE Dance theory mock! Because of you, you have made me determined, more determined than I have ever been before! I will get good grades, and although second best to dance, I will succeed at college and come out with a valuable 'Fashion Design' qualification.

I will never admit defeat - one day you will be killed; setting everyone free.

Goodbye from me.

X x x (Chloe Brookes) X x x

Dear ME,

You are so cruel. I've spent my whole life being told I lie, that I am wrong about my memories, I am wrong about what happened. That I lied about so much of my reality. And I've spent a lifetime proving I have not.

I even tried lying once when I was fourteen, screaming for attention; the shame was so awful I swore I would never do so again.

But how cruel you are, ME. How cruel. You crept up on me, and when my life was just getting right, finally you made a mockery out of me. You strike me.

How cruel you are. People in my life have lied, now you force me into the faces of doctors that lie to me. How do you prove to friends you are truly sick? They ignore your pain, because the doctor has already confirmed there is nothing wrong with you. Each doctor a new lie, each visit I lose a part of myself.

I find God. I start on the journey of proving them wrong. 20lbs of medical notes, CD's and reports each confirming the doctor's lie, but no-one listens. Still you lie. How cruel ME.

How cruel you are. You rob me of my career. You rob me of my use. You rob me of my purpose. You rob me of relationships. You rob me of friendship. You rob me of trust. And still you lie. Haven't you robbed me enough?

You rob me of my ability to have independence. You rob me of my energy. You even rob me in my sleep. How cruel you can be ME.

You put me in a sound-proof box and I am yelling; no-one hears me. You give me grief, as friends disappear one-by-one and each loses tears at my heart. You leave me with nothing.

Except my God.

You make a mockery out of me. You make me a liar. Even with proof. ME, you liar. You steal from me. You rob me. And you leave me empty, useless and rejected.

You are cruel to ME.

Dear ME,

I hate you.

I hate what you have done to me, to my life. That's because I have lost all sense of what life was like before you came along, I've forgotten what it is like to live like a normal person. I don't think you get it, do you? I was doing well enough without you. I made the most of every chance that came my way. I swam competitively, played hockey for my school team and was following my dream of becoming a dancer. You took all of that away and reduced me to a shadow of what I was before.

I'm frightened of you.

I'm frightened because I don't know what you will do to me next, when your next attack will come. Every time that I think I've got you figured out, you come and add something else to the list of symptoms that sends me down into a dark hole. Whenever I climb out of that hole, you are there waiting to push me back down every time. You are a bully.

I'm frightened of you because I can't face the thought of you being around me for potentially the rest of my life. I can't face the thought of even another day of your pain. I feel frightened about missing out on the most important things in my life. I get frightened at the thought that one day my children will have to care for me.

I'm angry at you.

I'm angry because you make it so impossible for anyone to work out why you are here and why you choose to mess up so many people's lives. I'm angry because you hide from view so that some people think that you don't exist, when all the time I can feel you there. You are so devious and so manipulative - you make people believe that we are lazy fakers because every time anyone comes near you, you become invisible. But when there is nobody is there, that's when you come out to play.

I'm angry because you have lost me so much that I wish I could get back. My job, my friends, my social life; the list goes on. Because people judge. People think I am exaggerating or even lying, because you choose not to show yourself, so they don't want to know.

But I am going to get you back one day.

I've still got my personality and a few friends who CAN see you for what you are. Whatever stunt you pull, however ill you make me, you can't take that away even though I know you try your best to. Us ME sufferers, we're stronger than you. One day we'll find a way of blocking your hiding place, of revealing you to the world. Then people will believe us and hopefully help us to get rid of you.

You won't win this one. I just hope that you haven't worn me down so that I never get to see you lose.

From Ayesha - your worst enemy.

Dear ME,

You hit me like a ton of bricks four years ago. But you lay in hiding all those years. You had them blame my mental state. You put me through four years of being poisoned by the worst medication that left me numb, drawling, and unresponsive to anything.

But you took a hold of me, and you sent me spiralling into a world of deceit. I didn't want you; I denied you so many times. Every time a new symptom or a new diagnosis was made, I would rejoice, see - it's not ME! But again you came back, and I hated you more each time.

How could you do this to me? Why? I will deny you every day. I won't accept you destroying my body and I will push you away at every chance I get.

I don't want you. This is my body and you can't have it. You may affect my short-term memory and I may not remember what's for dinner, or where I put my glasses, or put plates in with socks. But you will never take my memories; you will never take my joyous times I've had. I will hold on to them and remember the good times. And the lessons I've learnt from abuse. You can't have them. You can have my liver, my spine, my brain, my joints, you can inflame them all you want, but you won't get me.

You have altered me, but I am stronger than you and you will not defect me. One day you will answer to all the damage you do to twenty-one million of God's people.

I won't let you rob me of a life, as best as I can. And I will kick your butt!

From me...

Dear ME,

You turned my world upside down, and not in a good way. I lost all but a couple of my friends; why would sixteen year olds want a friend who can barely get out of bed? And when they do get out of bed has to use a Zimmer frame or wheelchair to get around? The world spins around you carrying on as normal, but you're stuck, peering out through the window, watching everything go by, wishing you were outside.

The pain you caused me I can cope with, it's the pain you caused my family. They had to watch their daughter, granddaughter, sister go through hell. They had to watch her crawling across the floor, struggling to brush her own teeth. For my seven year old sister, she had to push me in my wheelchair, she had to get me things when I couldn't move. I should have been taking her out, spoiling her with treats and showering her with everything she wanted, but I couldn't do any of that.

I lost everything that was important with me.

But I am grateful, because without having you I wouldn't have the life I have today. I would be carrying on like every teenager, taking a lot of things for granted and not stopping to appreciate what's around me. You have given me time to watch things happen, to step back and realise what's important to me. You have made me closer to my family and made my family so much stronger - yes, you did it in a rather unpleasant way, but you still did it. You gave me true friends who I know will be there for me no matter what.

I can think like this now because I am beating you, I am getting stronger every day. I still have a long way to go and you still give me reminders that you're still lurking in the background, ready to pounce if I do a fraction too much, but I have learnt to control you. You no longer have a hold on me. I believe that with every bad thing there is an equally good thing, take positives from the negatives. You made me grow up before my time; I had to mature overnight to become strong enough to deal with everything you were throwing at me. But I don't regret anything.

Yes, if I had the choice, I wouldn't want to feel like this and wouldn't want to have gone through all of this, but look, I don't have that choice. So I will take the positives from these last five years, and I will keep taking the positives from everything you throw at me because I'm not giving you the satisfaction of getting to me, and breaking my happiness. You have made me into a strong person, you have made me appreciate the small things that are all around me, you have changed my life. Some people might not see how it's changed for the better but I really am the happiest I've ever been, and making achievements that I never dreamt I could.

I'm sure we still have many days, months, years together, but I will keep growing stronger and know that with everything you throw at me I will take the positives, and one say I will be able to say 'I've beaten ME'.

Sophie.

A letter to my brain!

When you were well, you served me amazingly really. I took you for granted. Your thought processes worked in an instant. I didn't know you existed until one night when you said you weren't going to do this anymore.

I remember that day when I was overcome by fear, dread and a general loss of function that was totally alien to me.

From that day on to this you have only occasionally served me with reasonable function.

The tricks and games you like to play with me are like having a mind within a mind. You think it's funny when I can't remember things that are familiar. It must be hilarious to you that when I go to bed I lie awake for hours without sleep, with a brain that's racing away - but you're saying 'ha ha, no sleep for you tonight, but I might give you some tomorrow night'; but when tomorrow night comes you say 'oops - I was only kidding'.

Many times you think 'I'll put him in fear now, raise that adrenalin, ah, yeah a perennial panic attack, that would be fun'.

Then when I hit back with a reasonable spell, you say 'depression will sort that out or maybe OCD, or maybe a bit of both, yeah that's what I'll do next'.

So, Mr, you're thinking 'you're going through a good patch, I think a few seizures will put you in your place' and yes, the daily battle continues.

Nigel

Dear body,

I look in the mirror and feel let down by you. Surely people in their twenties shouldn't have bingo wings or so many wobbly bits? I'm too young for boobs to head south and too old to have a zit of such epic proportions, but you seem to disagree and bless me with these qualities.

Despite this, I think my body looks OK and after all, beauty is only skin deep. The wobbly bits aren't my issue with you - why did you have to let me down so much by turning against me? I'm sorry I spent time with someone with glandular fever when I was eleven, but I think it's more than time you got over this, let me be me, not someone with severe ME.

Being confined to bed for twelve years is no fun, nor is the level of pain you successfully manage to spread everywhere. Although I must compliment you on your wide range of neurological symptoms; it's an impressive array and could fill a text book on what can go wrong but please, do me a favour and go be in a text book and leave me the hell alone.

I appreciate that you, my body, does co-operate with me more than you used to. Thank you for letting me sit up after five years of being stuck lying flat, will you consider walking again soon?

I'm looking in the mirror, and aside pale skin and the dark eyes looking back at me, I really can't see you at all - although I can't see the bubbly, happy person I am either. You do a great job of hiding beneath the skin, it's no wonder so many people don't believe how ill you make both me and my friends with your presence; you even took my good friend's life.

Dear body, please release me from the prison that is you, let me get on with achieving my hopes and dreams, let me walk and dance, oh, and if that's not too much to ask, please take away the epic zit.

Yours faithfully,

V

A letter to my wheelchair,

Ours is a love hate relationship! Without you I am confined, restricted. You enable me to take part in life, visit places, shop, go out with my family. You expand my horizons but still I hate you!

Because of you no-one sees me anymore; you mask my personality, my intelligence and my abilities. People look past me or look down on me, people who knew me before this illness avoid the embarrassment of acknowledging me by crossing the street, or struggle to find something to say. You are the physical manifestation of my illness and I hate you, but without you I would be so much less.

Xx

Dear ME,

Compared to many of the amazing people I know, you haven't been in my life that long. I have 'only' been ill since January last year, but that hasn't stopped you from wrecking my life.

You have made me miss the past sixteen months of my education. Before you came along, I was on track to pass all my GCSEs, then go on to college, then uni, then get a job doing something I loved. Now I'll be lucky to get any qualifications – I can manage two hours of tuition on a good week – and my entire future is up in the air. I have so many questions, fears, anxieties, thanks to you. I don't know if I'll be well enough to go to college. I don't know what happens if I'm not well enough.

I'm lucky if I see my old school friends once every couple of months. It is a huge effort to go out, and when I do, I have to rely on mobility aids. No-one can tell me whether I'll be ill for a few more weeks, or months, or years, and it is the most awful feeling not being able to rely on your own body to work like it should.

It's not just me who has been so heavily impacted by you, ME. My mum has to look after me, take me to my appointments, comfort me when I'm crying because of how awful it all is and so much more. I rely on her and my siblings to do all the things I don't feel well enough to do. If I want to go round the supermarket, I have to be pushed in my wheelchair. No fifteen year old wants to have to depend on other people so much. You have ruined my education, my friendships, relationships with family members and much more. And the scary thing is, I am one of the luckier ones. I know people who are housebound, some bed-bound, yet manage to keep fighting you every day.

It is so unfair that you can just come into people's lives in a flash, and then we never know when you will leave. I hate you, ME, and I wish you didn't exist, but I know that one day I will be able to do all these things again, and one day we will find a cure.

Freya.

Dear my ME,

You stole my life, and for the last fifteen years I have been trying to figure out a way to accept and deal with the half-life you have left me with.

I was ten years old, giving it my all, practising six hours a day to become the next biggest star in the ice hockey world. I passed my rudimentary grades with ease, and sailed through to the next level. I was invited to join the team, but you took that moment to strike my strong body down.

The next year I had lost all of my friends (well how do you explain these things to children?) and I was bed-bound. Never had I experienced such tiredness, such distressing pain. Everyone told me to get over it, that I wasn't trying hard enough. You knew they would, you made all of my symptoms invisible, and who will believe a sick child who looks well?

School said maybe I was struggling with the work, or was it attention-seeking behaviour? You stayed with me. My father left shortly after, he never gave his opinion. You stayed with me. My brother, once the biggest influence in the family, was suddenly small and overshadowed by you. He followed in my father's footsteps shortly after. You cast him out, and you stayed with me.

My mother, well it's hard to say what she felt. She cried a lot, I could hear it in her voice, though the light was never on bright enough for me to see her face. She had to work three jobs to keep a roof over our head, and that meant leaving me alone, alone except for you. You stayed with me.

When I cried, it was you who was making me cry. The pain, the agony, the confusion.

When I tried, you struck me down harder than ever, intent at forcing me to live within these pathetic limitations, like a cage only I could feel.

The years passed slowly. Only those who have stared at the same four walls for years on end, sometimes by a candle flame's glow and later by the light of a mobile phone could possibly understand. The sun hurt my eyes too much for me to see the sky. It was lost to me. You stayed with me.

When everyone said I was a faker, your presence reassured me of my truth.

When everyone said I was exaggerating the pain, you made me scream, tears rushing down my face, arms and legs still but flailing inside. You stayed with me.

Now it has been fifteen years, and I reflect often on our friendship.

You erased shallowness from my world. You made me fight for every second of enjoyment. You made me suffer for my efforts. And still, though I think I have learnt all the lessons there are to be learnt from you, you stay. You stay with me. You remain holding the key to my life.

But I am breaking free from you; one rest at a time, one well planned out activity at a time, one dose of painkillers at a time. One day, I have to have hope, we all have to hope, I will be free from you. But you have affected my life so completely, that even if I ever recover health, the memory of you will stay with me forever.

But for now, you have made me tired just by writing about you. I can tell you want to stay with me.

An ME sufferer

Dear ME,

It's through tears raining down on my keyboard that I type this. I write on behalf of both my mum and I as you have affected us both equally - whilst I suffered, she cared, she worried, she did everything I should have been able to do for myself.

Most days I don't mind what's been taken from me; I've taken it in my stride and it's made me stronger, it's made me appreciative, it's introduced me to fabulous people. But what REALLY bothers me is what my mum has been robbed of. For five years she's had no life of her own so as to be my taxi, my nurse, medical secretary and spokesperson - all whilst continuing to work. She's said 'no' to so many opportunities of her own to be there for me and that's what guilts and upsets me most of all.

I remained determined, dedicated to my studies whilst everyone around me picked up the pieces and picked me up all the times I collapsed. Without my mum I wouldn't have even been able to get to the end of the garden, let alone the whole way to school. Twelve GCSEs, sixth form and art foundation later, yet still doctors tell me I'm 'lazy' and 'not trying'.

A teacher made me climb three flights of stairs when I could barely walk because 'there was nothing wrong with me'. I arrived at her door and fainted at her feet. The same teacher told me 'nobody would care if I was ill on the day of the exam'. I've been ill on the day of every exam I've ever sat. Another teacher told me the only reason I had ME was because I didn't eat breakfast, when I couldn't physically eat at all, at any time of the day.

Hours and hours, adding up to weeks and weeks spent in hundreds of different waiting rooms. Seeing doctor after doctor, consultant after consultant, being dismissed as 'mad', 'mental' or 'making it all up' more often than not - is it really any wonder at all that I developed a phobia of health 'professionals'? Being told I 'wanted to be ill' repetitively - can you really find me a single teenager who WANTS to lose the ability to walk, talk and eat?

A doctor told me 'my mum was making me ill' when my mum was the only person trying to make me better. Another doctor told me only 'sad, middle-aged women get ME'. I'm not even twenty; I sincerely hope this isn't middle-aged. And another doctor told me I was 'killing myself' by not moving enough. And yet another doctor shouted at me 'YOU'RE GOING TO HAVE A HEART ATTACK'; I'd never even spoken to her in my life.

Waiting years in constant physical pain for some actual help, all I've had is endless offers of psychiatrists, because it's easier to assume that a teenage girl is just stressed or depressed - I've never once even had a bad thought, but in all honesty would you blame me?!

Emily x

To this illness, ME,

    Broken-hearted me.

ME, you wrench my heart in two. Perhaps you think it's because you have shattered my life, put it on hold like some deadly pause? Or because you tear apart my body, trample my emotions, send shards of fear through my soul? Horror, pain, desperation... what word can I use to sum it up? There is none that describes the magnitude of such suffering.

Oh yes, ME, it's because all of the above, but there are more reasons. I also cry because of the others. The ones alone in this nightmare. The children. The youngsters. The artists. The unfulfilled rock stars. Their potential quashed and beaten into the dust. The waste of talent, snatched away before it can bloom. They are so much more than this illness. You have deprived the world.

They, all hidden away, longing to live, striving to improve, fighting despair, but so often thrashed back to their dark beds of sickness. So lonely in their grief, for no-one can understand their misery, or feel their heartache. Not totally. I've been there, am there still, but time and disease has dulled my memory of being so young.

I lost part of my youth to this illness as it descended at age twenty-eight, and that grates upon me, but there are those who don't even begin their life before ME takes it. They watch time tick, and yearn of what they might be. So unsure of how things will turn out, yet still they hope.

The unfairness is like a blow to the stomach, sickening and unreal. For that I am angry and for that I will weep.

xxxxx

Dear ME,

I don't know what I have done to you to make you treat me this way. I am bed-ridden and can't sit up for more than a minute anymore. I haven't walked freely since 2006 and haven't walked at all since the beginning of 2010.

I can remember so clearly the last day I crawled up the stairs that year. The last time I was able to have a shower, sat in my specialist shower chair with a carer washing me. Now it's just a flannel in bed that gets me clean.

I have had carers since 2007. And I dearly love them. But I want to be free. I want to wash myself. Shower every day. I want to be beautiful, wearing my favourite dress and heels, standing up instead of lying in bed. I want to go out my front door, to walk into the beautiful sunshine instead of seeing the sunshine shut away from me as each person leaves the house, leaving me in my prison cell, my punishment for a crime I can't remember committing.

I can't understand why I am living the life of an aged, dying woman at the age of twenty-eight. You've taken years from me; you've taken my dreams from me. And hope is a word that breaks my heart now. Dreaming breaks my heart. Longing breaks my heart. And every day the little hope I have fades.

But you won't beat me, you won't completely break me. Because even in the midst of my suffering, even in the anguish you can't destroy me; I will sing, I will create, I will live from this bed and let a beacon of joy rise up out of the ashes and I will win this war, I will win this fight.

And even if I never leave my bed again, no-one will ever say I gave into your ways.

'My health may fail, and my spirit may grow weak, but God remains the strength of my heart' (Psalm 73 vs 26). I have weapons ME, and I am not afraid to use them.

Love, Gemma x

Dear ME,

    Where did I go, what happened to me? I am not the person I used to be. Full of life, vim and vigour, now an almost broken figure.

Exhausted, fatigued, in constant pain, only tiny remnants of my past life remain. I long to sleep through the night, awake in the morning feeling refreshed and bright.

Unable to think or concentrate, my mind is in such a state. They call it brain fog, I can see why, head full of dark clouds like way up high.

Each day is a struggle, tasks to juggle, simple things like washing and dressing, exhausting, leading to depression.

Relying on others for simple things, only frustration and sadness it brings. Having to ask for a cup of tea, what the hell happened... ME.

From me.

Dear ME,

Well, where do I start? My life has become a whirlwind since you began to creep into it. I could never have imagined at my physical peak, I'd get struck down and my life would never be the same again. You've taken my teenage years from me. I'm somewhat of a daydreamer, so from an early age I always used to imagine my life - the things I'd do, the goals I'd achieved, the life I'd live. That was my first mistake; it's always the image of how things are supposed to be in your head that messes with you. I think that was the hardest thing, coming to the realisation that I had to get over what wasn't going to happen, at least not the way I thought. When you're caught between what was and what is yet to be, your mind fighting to get out of this prison you have put my body in.

You soon made my days consumed with lying down, my bones aching, my muscles weakening. My strength evaporating; I couldn't do the simplest of tasks without help, like getting changed or cutting up my food. The feel of touch, or noise could physically hurt my skin at times. I lost my concentration, the ability to string my thoughts together to put them into words. I became intolerant to dairy foods, getting into a cycle of eating less and less, becoming more and more rigid and restrictive in case of the consequences. You took every part of me I thought I knew and changed it; you changed me. All I could do was watch my life pass me by, frustrated, alone, confused and in despair. It wasn't long until I became absent from life, absent from the people I love. You took away parts of my personality; my confidence was at rock bottom. I was scared of the world and all that was in it. Every day with you was another day that you chipped away at me - mind, body and soul.

That's when that day happened. The day I'll never forget, the day I thought I was broken. My specialist made the decision that enough was enough - I needed to be admitted to hospital to be tube-fed and get me stronger. I couldn't walk at this stage - all I remember from that day is my dad trying to talk to me on the way back to the car, but it took all my strength to focus on taking each step back to the car. That's when he lifted me in his arms, both of us sobbing. Every day I could see you were making me break my parents' heart. You were tearing us apart - they wanted me to be better so badly, I just wanted it all to stop.

I spent around three months in hospital; I came out the other side of the 'dark period' you put me in. I was regaining some strength to walk again, putting weight on and seeing a psychologist for the depression and anxiety I was now fighting. I was becoming myself again a little more each day with the love and support of those closest around me. There is definitely no quick fix; I'm still taking my time now. There are always ups and downs. I'm still to this day using a wheelchair to be mobile outside the house, a walker inside along with other aids to help me. BUT I have the determination now that I didn't have back then. I will never allow myself to feel that helpless again because I know now that you can never break me. I will not give in, the mini-victories I achieve along the way outweigh you, because they remind me there's a life to live and a future to be had. I know now not to look for the end date of this, but instead I have to manage you, and to manage you I have had to accept you.

I don't know when or if I will ever be rid of you, I think you'll always be lurking in the darkness somewhere trying to remind me of my limits. But now I see that you do not define me. I will take control over you, I will accomplish my dreams when and which way I can. I've definitely learnt that it doesn't matter how long or the method of getting there, because once you do get there, victory is all the more sweet.

Over the last year I've started to achieve things I never would have imagined back then. I'm completing my Psychology A Level, I went on holiday abroad, I even went to a concert! All having their consequences, all having their restrictions - but none of that takes away the hope of a better tomorrow.

I'd love to wake up one day and not have you there. I can't actually remember how it feels to be a 'normal' person. To do an activity and not feel you there, to live complete and utterly in the moment. To feel ultimate spontaneity and not think of the domino effect of my actions. To have a day where I'm not scared of the world. One thing is for sure though; I refuse to be accepting of merely existing. I want to live the best I can within my limits.

Although now I do appreciate the little things so much, which I probably wouldn't if I had been a 'normal teenager' and for that I'm grateful. I know I have a lot to be thankful for. The value of family, friends, sunshine, laughter but most of all the value of life. I will continue to fight you every day in hope that one day I will be free. You may have determined my past but the future is all mine to play for...

Becca.

To the illness ME,

    How you have changed me.

You've made me suffer, filled me with terror of the next moment, left me scarred and traumatised. You've destroyed my view on life, changed my whole mind-set, turned upside down my belief system. You've wrung me dry of faith, contentment, trust, gratitude, joy. You've left me unable to smile. Stillness forced upon me. My only view of the ceiling, that's when I could bear any light.

You've left me angry, discontented and unhappy. Disappointed in my body, my associates, and the medical profession. I didn't know I had a temper, could be so horrible, could feel so selfish. I now swear.

However...

You have given me new skill sets, new interests. I've discovered new loves - extreme sports (to watch, not to do you understand), trick shots, knitting, crochet, beading, cross-stitch, nail art... oh my, you should see my nails! Computer skills, touch-typing, YouTube, Facebook; all things sitting down. I have made videos on chronic illness, I can identify a birdsong I hear from my bed, I'm a master architect in the world of Sims 3, and look! I can also write a thing or two.

I have developed patience, empathy, appreciation. I have slowed to a pace where I see more. I have the time to observe.

I now listen, the only ability I had left at times. I hear sounds more... water, wind, rain, sea, a crackling fire. Wolf howls, whales, crickets, jungle noises, frogs in rain, frogs by a stream, frogs in the summer, every nature scenario in MP3 format. Laying there, picturing it, pretending I was by that lake, deep in the ocean, among the dawn chorus.

Music, audiobooks, Amazon, online shopping... the wonderful world of the internet.

And the people I've met... those with ME and those without. Brave fighters, ones who have died, ones who have recovered, inspiring and motivating. Artists, musicians, writers... unending talent often relatively undiscovered, but also unspoilt.

Canadian composers, Swedish lyricists, American Guinness World Record holders, a Russian pedigree cat breeder... it's incredible who one meets when confined to one's bed.

They, entertaining me, encouraging me, making my world larger. Giving me distraction from my unendurable existence. How thankful I am to them all; they will never realise the good they do.

And I met my man through my ME *blush*. My soul mate and loyal fellow sufferer. Sharing my best times but also my worst.

Am I grateful for this illness? No, not really. Would I do it again? Not on your nelly! Yet, I am grateful for what I have achieved, the fight in me I've discovered and the determination I never knew I had.

ME, I won't thank you but I am telling you now, I will beat you and, though changed, I will come out better for it.

From Miranda Brewster, an ME sufferer since 2001

Dear ME (Myalgic Encephalomyelitis),

You turned my whole life plan upside-down in 2001. For this, I will never forgive you. Did you not think having severe glandular fever was torture enough beforehand? No! You chose to attack me and rage throughout my body, causing indescribable suffering without a day's rest ever since. I may be an adult, but my trusty Winston Bear has been with me since the beginning of this horrendous journey.

Getting the diagnosis of you - ME, on 17th July 2001 should have been a relief, knowing why I wasn't getting better and where treatment options were discussed but no, I was left to feel confused and to 'get on with it!'

Years later this is all too often still the case, not just for me but for so many ME sufferers.

I've learned to speak up more for myself and ask for help in a variety of situations, but the sad fact is even now there is still no cure for you (yet!). I have tried some treatments available and I will continue to look into different options, but all I ever see are what I call 'management techniques'. Although these are better than nothing at all.

You interfere heavily with my social life. Most days it being non-existent.

My beloved job in care with deaf young people with additional needs, squashed to nothing. I'd give so much to be well enough to work in a similar role again. I will always hope. You will never take my 'want and need' for life.

Medications barely touch the pain or the many other debilitating symptoms; the secondary anxiety and depression causes me, at times to feel trapped, consumed and desperate. The exhaustion I feel is beyond any explanation and the effects of any activity (where possible) appear any time after, even days after and last for weeks (Post Exertional Malaise - PEM).

ME - I would not wish you on my worst enemy. You are a living hell each and every day.

The devastation of ME cannot simply be imagined by non-sufferers. Family and friends often find certain aspects difficult to come to terms with and cope or understand at times, but they too suffer. Many lives are affected by your evil.

Sadly, you cause a lot of ignorance and misunderstanding. Being told I look well does not make me feel fine. I know people are just trying to make me feel better, but if ME wasn't attacking me I'd certainly look a lot 'better' for sure! I'd be able to look after myself. Plus, I'm seen by few people the days I'm looking even worse because on those days I'm too poorly to leave my bed or home.

I love life but I hate suffering with ME; you stop me living my life my way.

I gradually feel parts of my life are being chipped away to ME. How could you be so cruel? You won't win. You'll never take away my sense of humour when I do random things like mumble a sentence of words that don't even exist or make sense, yet I know what I mean! I occasionally even enjoy some of the vivid dreams you give me when you allow me to actually sleep! I hate being unable to wake up from them but I'm sure I could make some brilliant films, if I were well enough of course!

I have met some amazing ME friends (face to face and/ or online) who I will always appreciate.

I want to continue off-loading how I feel about you but now I need physical, mental and emotional rest. No words will ever be enough to describe the true extent of what you really are!

ME - A very real disease and disability.

From ME.

(Michelle Edmonds / Meesh-Mouse) xxxx

Dear ME,

I would like you to know that although you have inflicted yourself upon me, affected every aspect of my life and caused me high levels of pain and distress, you have not and will never defeat me.

I have the most wonderful friends, who have given me the strength to fight you. I cannot fight you physically, but I can fight you by remaining positive, by holding on to hope, by finding ways to work around you, by managing you in such a way as to minimise your effects as much as possible, to find creative ways to follow my dreams despite you, by taking good care of my body, giving it the right nutrition and plenty of rest, by patiently waiting until you realise you can never beat me and eventually leave.

And I find the strength to do all of this with the help and support of my wonderful friends.

I have a friend who knows my condition and all of its symptoms as well as I do myself, who completely understands it and always believes me, never thinking I am over-exaggerating, never getting cross when I have to cancel plans. She makes plans which are ME-friendly to include me, always keeps an eye on me to make sure I'm okay, and can tell by the slightest change in my expression or posture when the pain or exhaustion has become too much, even before I have registered the fact for myself. She doesn't always understand why I push myself beyond my limits but loves me anyway and accepts my decisions.

I have a friend who understands my illness in detail. But the greatest element of our friendship is that she has always treated me as the exact same person as before I was ill. She realises my limitations of course, and would never ask me to go above these limits. But I asked her to push me in my wheelchair to go out; she took it in her stride, didn't ask me a million questions about why I need it and how I feel about it, but agreed and moved on to other normal topics.

Which is exactly what I needed. I feel I can truly be my real myself, she sees the real me underneath the ME. With her I've never felt like an ill, disabled girl; I can see myself through her eyes as the same girl I always was, who just happens to be ill.

I have a friend who will listen for hours without complaining; when I phone her and agonise over making decisions to do with my health, she will discuss different treatment options with me and never loses patience with me despite my indecisiveness. I know that she is always there for me, and though I've needed her, I suppose, less and less over the years as I've got to grips with managing my health, knowing she is there if I need her is support in itself. She tells me her news which I love and takes an interest in my life even though it's not exciting. When I go for far too long without keeping in contact she understands and never makes me feel guilty for my lack of energy getting in the way.

I have a friend who sends me funny text messages and quotes which remind me that she cares and make my day every single time. She is always keen to visit me and tell me all about her adventures which I look forward to and enjoy, and she can make me laugh hysterically, forgetting all about my health problems.

I have a friend with her own health problems who is able to relate to mine completely, who understands what I'm trying to say about my health even when I'm not sure myself. She gets me completely and always has time for me, making me feel like family; I feel more at home in her home than my own.

All of these friends help me to get through life with ME by being there for me, each supporting me in their own way and I am truly thankful for them all.

Then there are all of my friends with ME themselves, and let me tell you ME, you're not beating them any more than you're beating me so you may as well give up!

There are far too many of them to describe, but they know who they are. They amaze and inspire me on a daily basis, they fight you as I do, and they are determined to beat you in the end. I am grateful to you ME for this one thing; for bringing these truly wonderful people into my life - they will be my life-long friends.

Together we will learn to control you, sharing tips on managing the symptoms you cause, together we beat the loneliness you cause by befriending each other, together we fundraise for charities researching treatment and potential cures, together we raise awareness, together we support one another though the ups and downs.

And together we will defeat you in the end.

From me x

Dear Fibromyalgia,

YOU SUCK! For the last eight years I've dealt with intense bullying, job loss, non-understanding family and boyfriends who don't try to understand, and who refuse to commit to me because of you.

I've been called a liar, a hypochondriac, a cry baby, useless and a lot of other things.

To think I was a healthy twelve year old. Then, my little brother passed and I developed depression, then viral meningitis, then glandular fever... and you managed to stick your grubby little fingers into the spokes of my turning wheel of pain and sickness, and you got trapped in there forever.

I'm now a strong twenty-one year old. You almost beat me. But I finally started opening up and showing my parents the severity of my symptoms. I started not caring about what people said. I found a man who loves me despite the havoc you wreak on my body. I'm in a stable two-day-a-week job found through disability support services and I'm just making ends meet these days. But I'm here, and I'm a fighter!

The strongest people I have ever known are the ones that have gone through intense heartache and trauma and come through the other side. We may have scars, but scars are toughened skin over the wounds. We are strong because of you!

Sincerely (still not a fan of you though),

Elyse Williams, twenty-one, from New South Wales in Australia

To my body,

     I used to think you let me down; I used to think you failed me. You couldn't keep going when I needed you to. Didn't behave when I wanted you to. You would collapse and faint at the most inconvenient moments, bringing upon me such shame and distress.

You would throw up these symptoms, out of nowhere it seemed; so unnecessary, so unbearable, turning my life into one of confusion and despair. I completely lost my trust in you, began to hate you, fear you. Terrified of what you would do next. I needed to rely on you but you weren't there for me.

ME isn't a proper illness (or so I thought); you can't put this upon me. Choose something else if needs be, something recognisable, something I can biologically understand, see on the doctor's test, read diagrams about in a book.

Okay, I admit I pushed you when you weren't well, trying to be the master, not wanting to be dictated to by mere flesh, but you should have been up to the challenge. Others are, so why not you? Look at these rock climbers, these marathon runners... there's no reason why you can't do that. We can be whoever we want to be, achieve whatever we want to achieve, surely?

But now I see differently, I've now learnt a thing or two. One thing I know is that if I ignore you, body, you will shout louder.

You were desperately vying for my attention, crying out for me to stop, hailing me with symptoms. But still, I brushed you aside. It's only when you snatched the reins and ground me to a halt that I began to take note. Even then, in a state of shock I fought against you for a while, grieving for the loss of my life that you had torn from me.

Eventually, however, I began to listen, stopped to hear what you were trying to tell me. I now try to understand, to communicate. I want to know what you have to say.

So, I see you as a surgeon, one with a job to do. A job of a healer. That's what you're designed to do right? If I cut myself, I heal. If I catch a cold, I recover... and what surgeon would perform well if despised, criticised, constantly told they're not up to the job? Like a wound being picked at and hassled, any recovery process hindered or brought to a standstill.

So maybe, if I let you be, give you the environment you need, give you empathy, sympathy, compassion... rest, relaxation, nurturing... you can battle this disease inside me and maybe, who knows, but maybe, one day, you may even succeed in overcoming it.

X

Dear Professionals...

To the treating doctors who were at the start of my ME journey,

Good morning from me and ME. You may be surprised to hear that I have found ways to manage many aspects of my ME. I am at present doing really well, and this was with no help from you.

After years of being ill with ME, and also having the added burden of needing to recover from the various treatments you, as my mainstream doctors, chose for me when I was too ill to research and choose for myself, I have now managed to make good progress. This progress began several years ago when I finally realised that you, my mainstream medical practitioners, were not interested in trying to understand or help me as an ME patient. Each of you merely treated my individual symptoms as they arose with medications that were intended to mask my symptoms, but in fact had more side effects than actual benefits. It got to the point where both you and I were unable to distinguish between which were new ME symptoms and which were side effects of your prescribed medications.

I was also told by you, my doctors, to keep up with high energy exercising each day for a minimum of thirty to sixty minutes and to keep working full-time. When I suggested on many occasions to you that this regime was making my health worse, you prescribed stronger pain relief and told me I would lose more mobility if I didn't push myself through this pain and this fatigue. At this point I somehow found the strength and determination to continue with this regime, but at a price. During this time in my life I was left unable to participate in any other life activities outside of resting, working full-time and doing my daily exercises.

It was just a few months later that my body said 'no more'. I was now no longer able to function. Now, I spent most of my time in bed. I was housebound and unable to work/socialise or look after my family or home and barely able to take care of myself. The only time that I felt I was alive was during my many vivid dreams. I was so very thankful for these dreams as they gave me a life.

Thankfully, I no longer live my life through dreams as several years ago I found myself a wonderful group of holistic doctors who understand and know how to treat ME. I now have no need to take any prescribed synthetic medications or even any over the counter pain relief, and I know where I am with my ME health. Now, don't get me wrong. I do understand there is at present no way of healing the ME patient's body, but there are many alternative treatments that can help the ME patient to have a somewhat healthier body and mind.

I am now able to get out and about. I now look after my family and home. I also socialise and work a few hours each week. I am not going to attempt in this letter to give you the details of how you can help your ME patients as each ME patient will be different. But I do ask you as professionals to take the time to educate yourself. Your profession is an important part of our society and many of us put a great deal of trust and faith into the fact that you will have adequate knowledge and understanding of our illness. The number of ME patients worldwide is growing and many will be relying on you to give them the best possible care and treatments available - and this can only be done if you are willing to educate yourself and try to gain an understanding of ME.

Thank you, from me - an ME patient.

To my doctor,

You always think you can put your faith and trust in a doctor to make you better - you just made me more ill.

Couldn't you see what you were doing to me?! Claiming I had a major psychological problem and all my symptoms were in my head!

I was having to use a wheelchair by then! The day you were dragging me out of bed up and down the hospital ward, making me walk when I couldn't even stand properly. Did you think I wanted to be like that?!

You treated me disgustingly. No-one should have to go through what I did. I had such high hopes that I was finally going to get some help for my neurological condition when I saw you... but because of you I ended up so ill, I was bedridden for eighteen months.

Luckily my mum fought for me and we found someone who actually understood my condition... see, it wasn't all in my head after all!

From Alex.

Dear Dr T,

My doctor sent me to see you when I was first diagnosed because she admitted she knew very little about ME. After following your advice to ignore my symptoms and to keep going to school, my health rapidly deteriorated so I went from being 85% on the ME ability scale to just 10%. I had been in school only missing mornings before I came to see you, and I then declined to being totally housebound and almost bed-bound. I felt sick whenever I moved and could not have a conversation more than a few sentences long. Even digesting food was exhausting and any kind of education impossible.

My parents and I naively assumed a doctor would know the right advice. By the time we got the correct advice from the ME charities to rest and pace my energy, the damage had been done. Now that I am managing my activity correctly my health has been improving, but I am still only 65% on the ability scale. It is twelve years later and I am still recovering from your bad advice.

I currently volunteer for an ME charity which brings me into contact with other young people with ME. I have met several of them who have similar stories about coming down with ME. Those of them who receive the correct advice and the support they need are often better, or at least nearly back to normal, within a few years. If I had had that advice and support I believe I would have been better years ago. Instead, although my health is improving, it will still be at least several more years before I am as well as when I first came to see you.

We would have made a complaint about you at the time, but I was too ill and my parents already too busy trying to look after me. My parents were also concerned that you might contact Social Services. The letter you sent to my school telling them I simply was not trying resulted in them being very unhelpful and made my education more difficult than it already was. It was only when I had an understanding home tutor who managed to explain things to my school that things finally started getting back on track. It was such a relief when I turned sixteen and was finally safe from you contacting Social Services. I hate to think how much more my health would have deteriorated if you had caused me to be taken away from my family; not only the people who I love, but my support network. They were the people who looked after me and protected me from people like you.

The first time we saw you privately you were polite, but the second time when we saw you on the NHS you were very rude, aggressive and unprofessional. I was too ill to answer your questions and you would not let my mother say anything at all.

You made it clear you thought I was either school phobic or attention seeking. You thought there was nothing wrong with me. You did not believe ME was a physical illness. Your ignorance and prejudice has cost me twelve years of an illness I would not wish on anyone. All I ask is that in future you treat people who have ME with the compassion they deserve. Please ensure you give the correct advice in future to prevent this from happening to anyone else. I would have been far better off if you had done nothing at all rather than everything that you did.

Yours sincerely,

KL

Dear Dr Matthews,

How can I ever thank you enough, for what you have done for me? God lead me on a search for a lung doctor and as I pushed the enter key on the Yahoo search, your name was down on the list. The reviews you had were not glowing, but for some reason, Dr Matthews jumped at me. My primary doctor told me that this would be the last referral they would do for me; I had already gone through two others. I waited patiently to hear from your office, only to be told that my doctor had to make the appointment. But I decided not to get frustrated at yet again being bounced around, and I let go of that control issue I have concerning my health. Finally I received a call - an appointment in three days.

I never ran the scenarios through my mind this time. So many doctors, so many disappointments - I decided to trust in the Lord. I never ran through my mind my old primary doctor of over ten years yelling at me to see a shrink. Or the attitudes of the Emergency Room doctors. Or the fact that some doctors would ignore my requests, as if I had not spoken. I was a person trapped in a glass box, banging my fists against the glass and yelling as the medical profession walked by, ignoring me. I pushed that all aside - I did not have time to ponder on the outcome, I just trusted.

My appointment was 9:30am on a Thursday in December 2013. Armed with my spine diagnosis and my previous lung function test results, I just remember being calm inside. The nurse came and got me at exactly 9am - I hadn't finished the paperwork. She was caring, compassionate and so gentle with me. 'This is new', I thought and it surprised me. We sufferers scare the medical field, and sometimes I want to say 'you are scared? How about what I am feeling?' but I don't, I try to put them at ease with a joke or a smile. I was left in the room with my own thoughts, my thoughts centred on my personal problems mainly. Within a few minutes a kind, elderly gentleman came in - you had a black dickie-bow on. I don't remember making eye contact that first time. You sat down next to me and said 'what can I do for you?' I handed you my letters and test results and told you what I knew about the respiratory system - no muscle strength, no air, no inhale, no exhale.

No hesitation from you, Dr Matthews, you confirmed what I have been yelling about in my glass box for a long time. You wanted to do some tests. Neuroplumonary lung function test, MRI of the neck and thoracic, blood work, and a barium swallow test. You wanted to see if a decompression of the neck would be possible to help stop the damage being done to the diaphragm, whether you could delay the inevitable. I watched you leave with a sense of loss, but with a sense of overwhelming gratitude and it was like the weight of the last fourteen years was lifted. I was finally validated, I was finally being heard, I was finally worth someone's time, and I was finally treated with dignity. To explain that overwhelming feeling of relief was just so earth-shattering. As your nurse walked me around to monitor my oxygen level, as we passed you giving the orders to a nurse, you looked over at me; 'you will be getting a flu and pneumonia injection today right?' How could I say no? You had already explained to me that 'people with this sort of neurological disease are susceptible to flu or pneumonia, and in their weakened condition they don't survive'. As the nurse lead me down the hall, I cried heart-felt tears; the nurse looked at me, and I said 'I like him'.

The tests came through. I wasn't able to do the two and a half hour MRI, not without being put under. So I waited for them to reschedule. But no call came, and I had been told if I hadn't gotten all the tests not to come back to the appointment your office made a month later. When I called your office the nurse's attitudes had changed; cold, rude, distant, and hardly returned my calls. It took three phone calls and two letters faxed to speak to a nurse, who then informed me no MRI's will be done, that you wouldn't sign the order for it. That is when I knew for sure that for months I had been telling doctors I'm dying, but was met with 'you are thinking negatively', 'your oxygen levels are great!'

I got the report from the hospital from the lung test. I can read; I knew it said 30% lung muscle strength that was down 17% from six weeks ago. But on the report that another doctor had written there was no mention of this. If a nurse were to look at it, it would say there was nothing wrong with me, or if even another doctor looked at it, they would think the same, nothing wrong. I wrote a nice, polite letter that Friday asking if it had been overlooked maybe? No reply by the following Wednesday, and after years of frustration, I used the Medicare and Federal Patient bill of rights; but again I worded it politely.

The next day I received a phone call from the nurse; the doctor had done an additional note on the report. So right away I emailed the records department and got a copy. With great anticipation and dread, and fear and hope all rolled into one, and me reminding myself 'trust in the Lord', I waited. It seemed to take forever; I kept checking my email and each time when nothing loaded my heart sank. Then it came! It was password protected. As I watched Adobe open it with fear and excitement, my heart racing, I broke down and cried when I saw what the note said. FINALLY it was acknowledged on my medical records I HAD A MEDICAL ISSUE! I called my girlfriend over; 'see, see, see' I kept saying! Three and a half years of heartache, stress, anxiety, heart-breaking tears, being ignored, ashamed, disrespected, rejected, dejected, and treated like an idiot, FINALLY to an END.

My personal issues had come to the point of a Protection Order and Adult Protection services being involved, and I needed somewhere to be. It was three days until my appointment with you was due. The crazy ideas that ran through my mind; you wouldn't see me, it would be another doctor, they would cancel my appointment, that this was all a dream. I needed help getting into a hospice where my protection worker was trying to get me placed.

The receptionist at the desk was brisk and unfriendly when she asked my name and checked my address - I had to tell her I'd moved. I didn't make eye contact, as my head had dropped so much; I speak barely above a whisper these days. I struggled to sit down in the waiting area. I wanted to cry, but I held it in; I held no resentment or anger at the nurse's attitude towards me. She seemed impatient with me as I slowly walked to the doctor's exam room. I was told to put my bag in there and come with her; she wanted to take my weight. I walked slowly, struggling with pain in my diaphragm - it was hard to breathe. This was the most I'd put my body through for a week; I hadn't left the recliner in nearly a week. I didn't meet her eye contact, I kept my eyes averted. She was brisk with me, and I think I even heard her sigh in aspiration a few times. I was told to wait - 'the doctor will be with you', in not so gentle terms.

Alone in that room I sat, my chest hurting and I was exhausted. I pulled my purple covered Bible out and lay my hand on top of it and closed my eyes and praised God and told him I trust him, in whatever plans he had for me. I've no clue how long I waited - forty minutes? Finally, Dr Matthews, you walked in. We didn't need to talk details, we both already knew what was going on; in my hand I held the note that my protection worker had given me, the information that the hospice needed to admit me. Softly you asked, 'what do you have there?' I told you, and you said so softly 'we can certainly do that for you.' Tears welled up and I smiled at you. I asked you what will happen. You told me that soon I would need ventilation. I shook my head - no; no measures were to be taken. 'Okay' you told me, 'the nurse will be in soon and I will get this seen to right away, do you have your protection worker's phone number?'

As you closed the door, I put my head on my hand that was on my cane, and felt the feelings of gratitude that finally I was HEARD, someone cared enough, someone respected me, someone heard me, and someone was helping!

It wasn't the nurse that brought me into the room that came to see me for me to sign paperwork; this nurse was soft, compassionate, and caring. As I walked out I said to the nurse's back 'please tell Dr Matthews, thank you so very much.' She didn't turn around but said 'I will'. As I walked out of the office I had to walk past the 'Check Out' window. I didn't have a paper to give them; I never did even on my first appointment. A nurse who was stood chatting to the administrative assistant asked me as I approached the elevators, 'did they not give you a piece of paper for us?' I looked up and said 'no, they are arranging hospice'. With some pride in my voice. Not just dignity and pride for me, but for the twenty-one million worldwide that suffer, not only with this devastating disease but the stigma attached.

We won, this day - January 17th, 2014.

Be strong in the Lord
Never give up hope,
You are gonna do great things

I already know
God's got his hands on you,
So don't live life in fear
Forgive and forget
But don't forget why you are here
Take your time and pray
These are the words I would say

'The Words I would Say' by Sidewalk Prophets.

Thank you Lord, thank you Dr Matthews. Thank you for all the advocates out there fighting for cures and funding.

Sincerely,

Denise Thomas

Dear Doctor,

As you are new and refuse to come and visit me, I have decided to write you a letter to let you know exactly how this living hell has affected me. I was a normal, healthy baby until I reached the age of three. I then started to cause my poor mother to keep taking me to doctor after doctor with fatigue, sickness, unexplainable aches and pains.

All the doctors told her it was psychological and to send me to school whereby I kept collapsing and had to be fetched home. There were periods where I felt like a normal, healthy child and managed to work (having bouts of tonsillitis, flu and time off). Then in 2004 I began to grow steadily worse, collapsed at work and now have severe ME. Surely you cannot write this illness off as all in the mind when I have pushed myself all my life to the point of collapse, pain, fear of what is going on in my body? I cannot tolerate many foods, I have fever, swollen glands, vision problems, pain in my muscles and joints and it goes on. Please help me; I am losing the will to live if this is all I have to look forward to (now you're going to suggest I am depressed and prescribe something which I cannot take or do not need). I and all other sufferers need action and support, not ignorance. I am now fifty-one years old!

Yours hopefully,

Suzanne Hogg

To the nurses who saw me in 2011,

I haven't used your real names in this letter as I don't remember most of them, but I will never forget my time staying on your ward. However, I expect you've well and truly forgotten me by now. I had some lovely moments, despite being in hospital, with other patients and a few of you who were brilliant. But I also have a lot of painful memories from that time because of the lack of understanding - the fact that most of you weren't willing to try and understand.

I was admitted as an emergency, late at night after collapsing at home and being in an unbelievable amount of pain. My first memory of being in hospital is waking up a lot later than others on the ward, asking what was going on and one of you asking if I remembered.

Sonya, the first of you to be looking after me during my horribly long stay was fantastic and so helpful. I can remember her explaining what was happening and finding me some tissues. She was wonderful all day and was very reassuring when I was so scared. Sonya was brilliant throughout my stay - she always had time for me and listened, and I hung on to that so much. Others of you also were lovely at first and when I cried, telling you that my ME had wrecked my life, you reassured me. You told me that you didn't know much about ME but you'd look it up and that I would get my life back. Did you ever really look it up? Or did you just go on what you thought you already knew?

For the first few days, I couldn't have faulted you. You were friendly, helpful, reassuring and you seemed to believe me. But then you turned because I wasn't getting better. You started to push me beyond my limits; you used to ignore my pleas to let me rest because the pain and weakness I was feeling was literally paralysing. You carried on pushing me and forcing me to do things that were making me feel horribly ill, despite me crying and begging you to let me stop. And when I did them, you told me 'see, you *can* do it'. You told me continuously that I had a confidence issue and that I just had to put mind over matter. Do you know how hard that made it for me? Do you know that half the time you caught me crying was because I was so scared of what you were going to force me to do next? I had so many horrible effects from that; extreme payback, all of which you completely ignored. And then you wondered why I wasn't getting better. The things you'd say made it out like I didn't want to get better.

My physiotherapists worked really hard with me and were very understanding. After a while, I was just about able to go from lying down to sitting on the edge of the bed independently. I will NEVER forget the horror and fear I felt when one of you, Cat, came up to me one morning; you told me that we were going to go for a walk up and down the ward that day. You'd never looked after or spoken to me before and knew nothing about me - you just judged me from what you'd been told. I can remember thinking 'are you *joking*?' and then worrying all day because of the effect it would have. I didn't want to tell you how I felt in case you completely dismissed it; I just didn't have the emotional strength to deal with even more tellings-off. Cat, you made me feel so humiliated. I was suffering from a physical illness but you refused to believe that it was ever anything more than a poor attitude and I actually became scared of you and what you'd say or make me do.

I can remember one night when I'd been there for a while, we were discussing when I'd be going home. I had really hoped that you weren't going to be the one to come and discuss that with us, but unfortunately you were. You asked me where I thought I'd be in a week's time, and I told you that hopefully I'd be out of there. You then replied with 'no, see, your attitude is completely wrong. You WILL be home, not "hopefully" be home'. I would never wish this illness upon anyone, but at that moment I wanted you to feel my pain so badly. I desperately wanted you to understand. I wanted you to know how it felt to be suffering so much and to receive so little support from someone who was supposed to be looking after you. I tried from that point on to avoid you whenever I could.

I can remember one of you, Linda, telling me that I had to have a shower one morning. Now don't get me wrong, I'm all for washing my hair every day but it was so difficult for me at the time that I could only manage it every few days if I was doing well. I explained to you that I'd had one the day before and that I wanted to save my energy as I had friends coming in that afternoon. You told me that it was more important to work on getting better than it was to see friends. But do you know what? They were getting me better. It was every bit as important to see them as it was to sit in that stupid shower so that you could tell me that I could really manage it. They were keeping my spirits up, and considering how I was feeling at the time, that was really important to me. So what did you do? You put me in the shower and left me there. The call bell was out of my reach. I was crying and shouting but nobody came for ages. So inevitably, I'd been sitting up for too long and felt awful.

Another of you told me that my friends and my boyfriend would only come and see me for so long. That you felt sorry for my parents. At one point you tried to argue with me that I'd been walking up and down the ward socialising when I was first admitted – we all knew that wasn't true. You made it sound like I could just snap out of it. But don't you think that if I could, I would have done it a long time before? Do you seriously think that I wanted to be there? Do you know how horrible it is, to see the whole world moving on around you whilst you're stuck? I missed my own graduation whilst I was in hospital - do you think that I wanted that to happen? Do you honestly think that I would have put it on?

I tried to keep quiet and almost agree with you at times, I tried to appear grateful to you all, because I don't like conflict and certainly didn't have the energy for it. But let me tell you now - what you did hurt. It *really* hurt. It hurt physically, it hurt emotionally. I eventually left hospital and was so relieved. But I was far from cured. Your treatment, your inability to listen and your constant pushing made me really ill. I suffered so much when I got home, but luckily I had very understanding people who visited me at home and who eventually saw me make progress. And you never saw that; if you had, would you have even believed me anyway?

You seemed to have me down as a lazy, attention seeking child (even though I was in my twenties) who had the wrong attitude to life and would never get anywhere. But I DID get somewhere. I went back to work and got a place of my own. I still have to manage my ME, it hasn't gone away, but I'm working around it. I proved you wrong and that feels amazing.

And do you know what? My friends and my boyfriend never stopped coming to see me. They never stopped supporting me. Because they knew that I never had a psychological illness and they knew that I was fighting so hard all the way. I apologise now that you've had to spend so much of your time reading such a long letter, especially from someone you had very little respect for. However, years after being with you I am still so angry at you for how low, how pathetic you made me feel when I was fighting as hard as I possibly could. There were a lot of people who told me that I should have made a formal complaint, but I never did. Maybe I should have. I suppose I didn't feel that it was entirely fair because some of you were wonderful.

I found it incredibly hard to trust anyone looking after me for a long time afterwards. With family and friends, that eventually faded. But it was only after being in a different hospital a couple of years later, where I was listened to, believed and respected, that my confidence in health professionals came back. But even now, I still approach people with caution.

I just hope you never come across anyone with ME again; I was strong enough to survive your judgmental views, but they might not be.

From a patient who can't forget.

To the nurse who didn't believe me,

This is a hard letter to write because it means re-living the situation you put me in, re-living the hurt you caused me. I was in hospital, in the private room overlooking the park, do you remember me? Of course you don't, because you have hundreds of people coming in and out every week, so let's see if this jogs your memory a bit more.

I was in hospital because I couldn't walk; my legs had lost all their power. I could still move them yes, but I couldn't actually use them to walk because they wouldn't hold me up. I called you in using my buzzer because I needed the toilet and usually someone would push me in my wheelchair, or push my drip alongside so I could crawl in myself.

You came in and as I got down onto the floor you said 'what are you doing?' I explained that I couldn't walk and needed to crawl, so please could you push my drip along for me? You said you wouldn't do it and that I had to walk. I was shocked at this point, I really couldn't walk and I didn't know why you were doing this. You kept saying 'if I let you crawl then you're never going to walk again, you have to get up, and I will hold onto you and help you in'.

What else could I do? I was crying but you still made me get up. I collapsed twice on the way to the toilet but you still made me walk. You then told me I had to wait in there when I was finished, and call the buzzer so you could help me walk back. Once I was finished I rang the buzzer; I promise I did, but you didn't come, so I crawled back, struggling to push my drip alongside me, but I made it back to the safety of my bed.

You then came in five minutes later and said 'what are you doing? How did you get back here? You crawled didn't you?!' and made me feel terrible, went to test the buzzer and said 'well you obviously didn't pull it hard enough because otherwise I would have come.' You then left me in pain and sadness to try and get over that traumatic ten minutes.

My mum had only gone home for breakfast but when she returned she was faced with a traumatised daughter. Later that day I saw my physio who said I was under no circumstances allowed to walk, because when I stood up I blacked out. After that, I used a Zimmer frame to stand up for a couple of minutes at a time.

It wasn't my fault; I just needed someone to believe me.

Remember me now? x

To my OT,

You are meant to understand my illness but you all do is push, push, push. Nothing I do is ever good enough. I am proud and think you will be pleased with me as I have been going to school much more than before, but all you do is say I need to stay there longer, and if I feel ill I can't go home early. I can't get to sleep at night and you make me feel like it is my fault. You tell my parents to ignore me at night-time, even when I am upset and feeling scared and lonely. Luckily for me they ignore you! I am so tired but you say I still have to get out of bed and walk, even at the weekend after I have been at school all week.

I don't like coming to see you, it makes me worry what you are going to ask me to do next. My mum tells you I sometimes feel much worse but you tell us I just have to do more, more, more. You speak to my school and I worry they will be on your side and expect more of me too. I hear my mum and dad talking about you and that makes me worry about what you are going to tell us to do next. I think you should care more about the children who come to see you and try to understand what they are going through.

From Isla, aged eight.

To my fellow physiotherapists,

We know how much good physical activity can do for people, and using movement and exercise to improve function and wellbeing is what we do. So of course it's natural that we would want to use exercise and movement for people with ME. However, we need to stop and think and change our usual approach.

This is a group of patients who consistently report Post Exertional Malaise (PEM) – an increase in their symptoms if they do too much activity. Our treatments/ interventions should never make people worse, so we need to listen to what people with ME tell us and understand how little activity they can manage before bringing on the PEM in order to find an accurate baseline from where to start.

It's hard to believe what they tell us. How can so little exercise cause such an increase in symptoms? It doesn't seem to fit with everything we have learned from our work with other groups of patients. And until my son developed ME out of the blue, I certainly never believed it would be possible.

One of the questions included in the pages we were asked to complete at our hospital assessment asked if he could walk the length of a football pitch. He said yes, as he can indeed walk the length of a pitch without any problems. However, within two or three days, he would be confined to bed as a result of this seemingly small amount of exercise, and it would probably take him two to three weeks to get back to where he was before walking the length of the pitch. Again that doesn't seem right – to get a previously sporty teenager back to his previous levels of sport, surely we need to actively rehab him and encourage him to increase his activity until he is 'fit' again?

ME has turned my thinking on its head – there is research to show that patients with ME aren't able to reproduce exercise treadmill test results twenty-four hours after their first test, so how is our 'usual' approach of regular exercise to improve function and fitness levels meant to help?

We need to change our approach to people with ME – at present, 'physio' is often seen as a dirty word for people with ME who have been given over-ambitious exercise programmes, which have only made their symptoms worse. Patients are avoiding the very people who could help with the management of their condition. As physiotherapists we have a lot to offer people with ME through pain relief, advice on posture, advice on activity/ exercise, including the exciting work around analeptic exercise coming out of America which aims to restore functionality lost through inactivity, give patients a sense of control over their illness and, hopefully, improve the quality of their lives.

As a profession we need to ensure we are improving the health of all our patients – treating conditions we are competent to treat, carrying out thorough assessment and regular review of progress, and adapting exercise programmes as required. I believe that physical activity does have a role to play in the care of people with ME. But this must be individualised for each patient rather than adhering to a rigid protocol and start from the level that the patient is at, even if that seems an unbelievably low level.

We can't risk making any of our patients worse with our therapeutic interventions. If patients are telling us that they feel worse after doing any activity (however small) why should asking them to do more exercise make them get better? We certainly wouldn't ask a patient with a musculoskeletal problem to keep repeating the movement that causes an increase in their joint or muscle pain, so why ask a patient with ME to do more activity, when even functional activities like washing, showering, shopping all cause an increase in their symptoms?

We owe it to all our patients to ensure that we are up to date on the latest research for the conditions we treat, to listen to our patients as they describe what activity does to them and to ensure that we do no harm with our treatment/ interventions. We also owe it to our profession to ensure that we are seen as professionals who can help people with ME.

So please listen to your patient with an open mind, read the range of evidence about exercise for people with ME and provide your patients with therapeutic interventions that can support them to manage their condition. Our treatment must make people with ME better, not worse.

From a fellow physiotherapist.

Dear Man,

    I don't think it matters or in fact I don't care that I don't remember your name. I wasn't treated as a person by you and I therefore feel like I shouldn't treat you accordingly. But I don't do that, I address you as a man because I recognise you as a person despite what you did to me and the fact that you may not deserve it. Should I think that you were uneducated? Ignorant? We are all subject to hypocrisy and behaving in ways we later realise were not compassionate. But you were in a position of responsibility, of care, and it was not acceptable: morally, ethically, professionally.

Not only did you subject me to taunts and to the sarcastic bite of a bigoted mind, but you forced me to endure physical pain and more than those physical symptoms because I was too 'lazy' and was a 'liar'. I was a child. A sick child. Under your care. You victimised me. You waited until I was alone, vulnerable, unable to face you, to defend myself. You stood face-to-face with me and stuck in the knife. You were so cowardly, so cruel and callous. When I think of myself then as a child, I only see a detached child in my mind; I cannot believe that you would do such a thing. And then to take a career in a 'caring' profession. I wish you were the only person I had met who contained this specific paradox.

To tell a child who cannot support themselves, physically, mentally or emotionally, that they are making it all up, that they are holding us all up. That I was worthless, stupid. I was not stupid then and I am not stupid now. And yet even now I have problems with feeling believed. In fact I don't just have problems, it is a problem in my life now as an adult. I cannot move on because people like you, and you as an individual, made me feel that what I was experiencing couldn't possibly be true. Even when I was so physically ill I took an hour to get back after everyone else, subject to sly taunts and forced to make myself unwell for the satisfaction of your ignorance. To turn up at the van in a state of exhaustion and symptoms when I had spent over a year bed-bound in a state of living death. But I wasn't worth your compassion, or indeed that of others (who you tried to convince of my histrionic behaviour), or food for which I was denied for my lying. That such a person as myself would never get anywhere, would never be anyone because I was wrong and deceitful. As if you cared about specialist diagnoses.

Do you deserve this letter? I wonder if I should do it. Does this give you a power over me, which we establish you still have, by affecting me years and years after the experience and years into recovery? Yet I feel that in writing this I defend the woman I am now and I defend the girl I was then. It is not acceptable to treat anyone as I was treated. It is especially not alright to abuse your position of power to do this. To take a physically impaired small girl and intimidate from a position of a man both physically larger and stronger.

I could edit this letter, I could re-read and tighten the grammar. But I am not going to. It does not matter if this letter is not perfect or all that I could say. This is me now telling you, in this moment, that this was wrong. You were wrong. People who are compassionate, not people who understand or who are even informed, but people who are compassionate and empathise, who don't jump into conclusions, who don't abuse their positions; they will not judge me for writing this in one stream. I can't even, I don't even, want to go back to the full memory. Did you know that I once saw you in a coffee shop and I had to leave, because I felt that I didn't deserve to be there, that I had no right to that? Somehow my presence was disingenuous and I couldn't stay. In writing this now and realising that I shouldn't have left, I am still thinking in language that suggests I had to prove myself to deserve being there. I don't have to prove that I am ill anymore. With the condition that I no longer have I do not have to justify, but even with those that I do, I don't have to prove myself. To anyone. I avoided that coffee shop, I avoided that place, I avoided going out because I felt such anxiety that you or someone else who be there to judge me. To make a superficial conclusion on my truthfulness in the life I was then living. This went on for years.

You picked on someone who was vulnerable, who couldn't speak out. Just because I can speak out now doesn't mean that's the reason for writing. I write because I am for myself. This isn't for you. This is for me. That I do not have to feel this way anymore, that I will not let you affect me anymore. That not everyone is the ignorant, cowardly jerk that you are. You don't deserve stronger insults. I don't wish you ill and I would always hope that everyone is doing well. I want you to know that I believe in myself, in how I felt and how ill I was, and that whenever I am in doubt I will remember that you abused me, and that I know now that your opinion is worthless. I can't let my life be dictated by this anymore. I can't spend my days wondering and struggling to be believed, to be loved because I do not feel I am believed. I am trustworthy, I am honest, I deserve respect and trust.

Sincerely,

V

To the NHS ME Clinic,

      I looked to you for guidance; I looked to you for help. You were supposed to be the experts, my support. You were supposed to take my word for it on how I suffer, without question. Not doubting my sanity and calling in the psychiatrists like the doctors did.

I was desperate for your help, I needed you so much. You will never know how much I cried after your first home visit. My hopes had been so high. I didn't expect bafflement from you; I had enough of that from myself. You told me you had never seen someone so ill with ME, that my severity was rare. Yet I know so many brought down as low by this disease. Why don't you know this? You denied their existence.

You sent out your occupational therapist, specialising in the housebound, in the severely affected.

Not only did you leave me with confusion but you left me with a timetable, impractical and impossible. Go downstairs at 8.30am, it began, and make yourself toast. Then rest for fifteen minutes. Then go upstairs and wash. Then rest for fifteen minutes... fifteen minutes rest, fifteen minutes activity, day in, day out, that will see you right, will build your stamina. Spend time downstairs every day, you need to be upright and moving or your muscles will waste, you risk immobility syndrome, depression...

Dutifully I followed your advice, and pushed myself. I couldn't manage the 8.30am toast but every day for three weeks I forced myself to sit downstairs, when my body shrieked out for bed rest. I did your fifteen minutes, hoping, believing that somehow you were right, always knowing in my gut that you were wrong. My gut won out. In September 2011, any scrap of strength left me and I have been unable to go downstairs since. For that I blame you.

And then the lack of support, infrequent visits, brief phone calls every six months. Passing me on, referring me elsewhere, to a psychiatric ward, of which I've heard horrors. Eventually discharging me, as I had failed you by my lack of improvement.

Because we with ME don't fit into how you expect us to be, because we don't recover by your 'treatment', we are the ones in the wrong. Almost accusing us, blaming us, like we are messing up your records. Treating us like criminals.

Do you have your heads in the sand? Your minds in the clouds? Do you actually know that 25% of those with ME are confined to their houses, to their beds? Hidden from NHS view. Do you ever ask the sufferers what we need, how we feel? Not wanting to know of discoveries we've made or therapies we are willing to try?

So we write our own books, set up our own charities. We support one another, test and try our own treatments. Yet whatever the outcome, whether we are successful or not, ME Clinics - we will do this without you.

From one of your patients.

Dear Healthcare Professional,

     I know what it's like, you know, to be on your side of things. I've been that person who got frustrated with the patient that constantly pressed their buzzer, or kept asking for pain relief. I've been the person who made snap judgements based on how a person acts or their diagnosis. But I know now how much that hurts, because now it's me that has the diagnosis everyone makes snap judgements about, including you.

I want you to be able to see me. I want you to ignore that bit of paper that says 'Chronic Fatigue Syndrome' or 'ME'. I want you to forget everything you've been taught about what ME is or isn't and just look at me. I want you to know that I would never choose this, that being bed-bound and unable to work is not fun. Lying in bed all day got old after about two days and I just want to be out working and socialising and just being a normal twenty-two year old. You see, I loved my job. I loved taking care of the people who needed it most. I loved helping people to get better. And one of the best things I learnt as a student nurse is that a patient with a long term illness usually knows far more about their illness than you as a health care professional will know, and so the most important thing for you to do is listen. Except you don't. You look at me and you just see a diagnosis. You see a twenty-two year old in a wheelchair and you make a judgement. You tell me that a twenty-two year old shouldn't be on strong painkillers, or be in a wheelchair... and you're right, I shouldn't be in a wheelchair or on strong painkillers because most twenty-two year olds are off at university or travelling the world, not lying in bed in agony, but I am, no matter how much I wish I wasn't. I just want to ask you to see me, to look at me and imagine what it would be like if it were your daughter or your sister sat in front of you. Would you not do everything in your power to help make life better for them? Or would you just dismiss them because of the diagnosis they have, that from what you know about it means they are just a bit tired, or worse, making it up? Would you deny them pain relief that works simply because you've heard otherwise?

There is no other illness that I can think of where the only treatments that are available are harmful to patients, where they end up seriously ill as a result of following doctors' advice, advice that you gave me! I don't know of another illness where a doctor can refuse to see a patient because he has no interest in that illness. I wish every day for a different diagnosis, for attitudes to change, for proper biomedical research to be done, so that for once I'll be taken seriously by you. More than anything else I don't want any more people to suffer or die from this illness because healthcare professionals still believe that it's 'all in our heads'.

xx

A letter to those doctors that don't believe in ME,

Please listen carefully to what your patients are telling you... I too was once a doctor and believed the limited education that I received about ME, that this was a psychological condition - that somehow, for some obscure reason, thousands of people were imagining exactly the same symptoms and were using this as a way to avoid working! Really? Who in their right mind would chose to spend days on end lying in a darkened room? What benefit do they gain by being unable to get out and socialise, or take part in their hobbies and interests? Look more closely at your patient and what you know about their personality - is this a lazy, work shy individual who all their life has exaggerated any minor problem, or is this a previously healthy, active, striving person who has been struck down by a devastating, life-changing illness?

I know it can be difficult to make sense of the multitude of seemingly disparate symptoms and to believe your patient can one day walk to the surgery but the next day is bedbound, I fully appreciate that it may seem impossible that one person can have so many different pains and other symptoms, but please listen to me when I tell you that this illness is real... the overwhelming fatigue when you can barely lift an arm, the burning pains in muscles and deep aches in joints, the problems processing information like reading, thinking, simple maths, simple tasks and speech. The rapid pulse, light-headedness, breathlessness and cold extremities, the never ending sensation of coming down with the flu, the balance problems and other neurological symptoms, the Post Exertional Malaise which renders you helpless a couple of days after any exercise etc. etc. - the list of symptoms could go on and on.

Imagine what it must feel like to suddenly find yourself trying to manage with all these symptoms; what patients need is your support and understanding, not your disbelief. It is hard enough managing this illness with help and support, but imagine how much worse it must be when the one person you hope to get help from doesn't believe you!

Please listen to your patient with an open mind, read all the recent research which clearly shows this is a physical illness and give your patient the support and belief that they need.

Yours,

A former doctor.

For the attention of those in the medical profession,

> I couldn't get to the doctor's yesterday.

Sleep is like poison to me, and I've been increasingly waking up as if I'd drunk a gallon of Special Brew the night before. I shiver the way through the evening and then wake up boiling, even though the room is the same temperature. My mouth tastes and feels like it's full of salt, and my belly is like a balloon with the guts inside aching. The cold burn down both sides of my neck and down my throat is particularly bad when I wake. And that is just what happens when I sleep. To wake is to be in immediate distress.

From midday yesterday I was trying to organise going to the doctors, though I truly felt (and still feel) too ill to go. Before I left London Rd, they said they would be able to help me throughout the transition period, and I would be able to get help with things like getting to the doctors. So I rang them up, and was given the brush off by the assistant manager; she told me it was nothing to do with them now, and I must talk to 'Joanne'.

I rang Joanne, and was rudely told to go away as she was in a meeting. (Today, she came to see me and immediately spent ten minutes on the phone talking to someone else.)

I rang my doctor's to say I had to see them, but was ill in bed and had been discharged with no cash. They went to talk to Dr Riley, and came back with the very useful message that she would like to see me. Had nothing useful to suggest as to how I could do that.

I tried to ring the PALS 'service'. The number I had was out of date. Eventually I was put through to the hospital. The receptionist did not know of any direct number for PALS.

I told the hospital PALS woman what a terrible state I was in, how I had been contemptuously dismissed at A&E the night before, and left to find my own way home with no cash and no house keys. When I said I had been discharged with no cash and no way to get to my doctor's appointment, she immediately latched on to the opportunity of passing the buck, as does everyone else.

She told me that, contrary to what its name suggests, the Patient Liaison and Advisory Service is neither a service, nor does it liaise between patient and health service provider. 'It' is an unconnected diaspora of small departments, or delegated persons sharing only an acronym - each within its own discrete NHS unit. Nobody is in charge; there is no organisation, and no accountability.

So the buck was passed to another PALS; one for SEPT. This one rang me. Time was pressing as I explained my predicament. They said Joanne would ring, but she didn't. They also said PALS CAN'T liaise between doctor and patient (do they do anything at all?). It is, apparently, the CCG, that now liaises with patients. And so the buck was passed again.

I tried Rethink, and got a dead line.

I tried Penrose, but they don't 'do' health.

I tried PohWer, but nobody was available to advocate for me. This is another mis-named service.

So I got the CCG number, and, amazingly, I found someone who would accept responsibility! [Stand up Mrs S! Applause.] Mrs S, though she is officially designated 'Child Safeguarding Officer', took a great interest in my story, and even wants to know more. She was taking notes as I spoke, and she wanted to get the facts straight because the CCG needs to know what are the local deficiencies and unmet needs in their community, so that they can commission what is needed.

I explained that the root cause of all this was the lack of a designated diagnostic service. Without one, time-pressed

GPs and A&E staff can just stamp 'MUS' (Medically Unexplained Symptoms - thank you so much Prof. Wessely) on your file, and pass the buck to the psychiatric services, who, themselves, have no space, few doctors, and no idea what to do with the majority of MUS subjects - who are just victims of the system, and not mentally ill. They do, nevertheless, always manage to find an appropriately unprovable pseudo-diagnostic label with which to further burden the patient, and compromise his chances of obtaining medical services in the future. This label is lifelong and irrevocable: a life sentence; too often, a death sentence. It should be illegal.

Mrs S very kindly took up my case and phoned my GP's practice, and went to discuss the matters I had raised with her colleagues. She rang back and said the duty doctor at the practice was going to ring me.

Half an hour after I had missed my appointment, I got my call from the duty doctor. She said I had missed my appointment. I told her the whole story. She said Dr Elliot wanted to see me... [All sing: 'But, there's a hole in my bucket, dear Lisa...'] I tried to explain to her what doctors were for, and that it was them who were supposed to be providing a service to patients, and not the other way around. She said try the CAB. I said, not to worry, I'd just go away and die; and hung up.

I was left entirely without any avenue of help other than to further burden my sister and her partner and make them suffer with me, also with no way to help, and no avenue to get any from anyone in a position to do so.

I spent the evening and night shaking in bed, with scarcely the strength to get up for the loo. Even reaching out to pick up the notebook sent me into palpitations and set my whole body shaking from the effort of using my arm muscles (what is left of them.).

When I do get to sleep, it is a relief, and I have pleasant dreams, but I really do wake up as if someone has been filling me with poison. It is always a terrible shock. [I also need to rebalance the radiators, because the radiator in the hall is shutting off the thermostat before my bedroom gets warm. Cold air on my skin sends me into paroxysms, which can make getting out of bed dangerous.]

And so, for my ten o'clock appointment with my 'couldn't care less' co-ordinator. I was doubled up over my bloated belly and nearly in tears when I struggled down to open the door to her at ten-past-ten. As always, she completely ignored this, and breezed in to put the kettle on.

She'd brought a Department of Work and Pensions letter for me, and insisted I open it so she could see what it was. It was for my DLA 'overpayment' tribunal [incidentally, only due to another SEPT cock-up, in not informing the DWP when they sectioned me for annoying the NHS], but I said not to worry about that because I was ill, and might be dead by then - so what could she do to help me get the care I actually needed, rather than the interference she wanted to do as displacement activity in place of her nominal job? She made no apology for not calling me yesterday, even though she said PALS had called her about it. Then the phone rang, and she spent ten minutes in the kitchen talking to someone else.

When she came back to me, where I was still shaking, she did, at least, bring me some tea and toast. But she then sat playing with her phone, as she was having trouble setting the GPS to find the best route to her next appointment: 'I'm useless with technology.' She said. She has said this before, as an excuse for not keeping me in the loop via email, which has meant I've never known what SEPT is planning for me unless I find out by chance. I learned from Penrose, that she does, in fact, communicate with them by email. Despite this, mug as I am, I still tried for a minute or two to help with her phone.

Eventually, I got to relate to her what happened yesterday. She listened without the slightest trace of empathy or consideration for the position and predicament of her client. I got so exasperated by her callous behaviour, while I was sitting in an obviously distressed state beside her, that I made one last attempt to explain to her exactly what is meant by being responsible for someone's care. I pointed out to her that all that would have been needed to help me, in the whole of the time that I have been under the 'care' of SEPT, would have been for her, or anyone else in the organisation to pick up the phone and make a call on my behalf, to any responsible person in medical services, and explain that they could not help me and that my physical illness needed properly looking into.

They have already admitted that their 'treatment' was useless. They have even dared to 'suggest' that my best next step is to see the 'experts' (psychiatric of course) at a different hospital. These are the very people I had arranged to see over three years ago, before SEPT told the PCT that they could treat me locally, and blocked the treatment I had already had one introductory session of.

Joanne listened to all this in total incomprehension. She and SEPT could have saved me at any time in the last three or four years with a simple phone call, but no-one, from the cleaner to the CEO was willing or able to do so, or even to think that such communication between the physical and mental branches of the NHS was possible.

She stood through these home truths like a deer caught in the headlights, then said that I was being very rude and that nobody should talk to her like that. Then my 'carer', my only officially appointed representative, left me helpless, still cash-less, and in considerable distress.

I was still a bit puzzled as to why she'd come to 'see me' on a Saturday; only when I was left helpless and wondering what to do next, did I notice my sister's email. After ringing her and finding her not in, did it dawn that today is Friday, so I can still communicate.

I'm still in a lot of physical distress. I can't tell what is hunger and what is pain, but I have little desire to eat. I've had three packets of nuts, two bananas, three plums, a bag of crisps, and a small pizza since Tuesday, but I still find it hard to contemplate eating while I am in so much pain.

I'm copying this to Mrs S, and will ring her again when it's done. I pray that she may be able to help.

Yours,

Steve H

To the PALS officer of the local Clinical Commissioning Group,

I've just got off the phone from Dr P after a call from yet another uncaring and confrontational GP. I had tried to talk to you this morning, but spoke to someone else instead. She advised me to call Dr P and ask for a home visit. I was very wary of this, as they have been very cold and unhelpful to me for a long time - but I gave it one more shot, and the receptionist said she would get a doctor to call a telephone consultation.

This 'consultation' took the form of a disbelieving confrontation, with, yet again, all the emphasis being put on the belief that the patient is there to serve the doctor rather than the other way around. So, yet again, while I am in bed, almost too frightened to move, instead of being offered help I am subjected to the kind of sarcastic verbal bullying I am more used to hearing in a rowdy pub, as the prelude to a fight.

The doctor insisted on me going to see him no matter what, and again, pointed out that I had 'missed' the appointment with my GP, as if this was both my fault and something of a crime. He also said that I had not been to see them enough for them to get to the bottom of my problem, when they have done everything they can to put me off visiting them, have been brusque and dismissive when I have managed to visit - and never shown the slightest concern for my health, let alone willingness to actively participate in investigating it.

Having been pretty much forced to rely on the Walk-In Centre and the internet for advice, I am then told off for using them - by the very people who cause me to have to do so.

It was their unwillingness to help me that led to my having to rely on the deputising service and A&E, and, eventually, being dumped on psychiatric services and wasting another nearly four years of my life and a great deal of public money. And now it is abundantly clear that they intend to carry on where they left off. Where one would have expected at least an apology, all one gets is still more insolence and confrontation.

The NHS, as far as I have seen, is entirely suffused with the attitude that anyone who has suffered for a long time is OK to leave to go on suffering, no matter how bad it gets. I was again challenged to go in to see this horrible person, or go away and die. What could I do but put the phone down?

Please, can you find out if there is a better GP in town, who has real experience and interest in chronic 'physical' illnesses and wants to effectively diagnose them and seek cure? Or who at least has some compassion for the suffering of their patients, because I am ruing the day I ever had anything to do with the, utterly dreadful, Dr P.

Sincerely,

Steve H

To those who want to learn more about the battle for severe ME sufferers,

More nails in the coffin, for the 25% severely affected.

So, after a week in which I was, essentially, told by my GP to go in and see him on his terms or go away and die, my faint hopes were pinned on someone who had tried to help me with CBT before I was forced to abandon this avenue and accept what 'services' were available locally - leading to three and a half wasted years of psychological abuse and indifference to my steadily worsening health...

This someone has now risen to be in charge of a unit commissioned to deliver CBT services in the county. I had hoped that she/ he would prove to be an ally, and a useful contact. I had been led to believe, from the publicity surrounding the opening of a new 'CFS clinic' in the area, that potential clients for this clinic were to be assessed both physically and mentally, and that there would be a consultation with the 'experts' in charge beforehand. In hope of this 'second opinion', I had applied for this service, and sent in a number of blood samples. However, I had heard nothing more from the service, until, a few days before I was discharged from hospital, I was told by the shrink in charge that the service had turned me down. I was denied the chance of any face-to-face consultation with the clinic over my health.

It turned out that my acquaintance was the psych component of assessment for this new clinic. When I last met her/ he, she/ he seemed fairly open-minded, and I had liked her/ him. Now she/ he was as closed to reason as all the rest. When I tried to explain that, after three and a half years, I had given psych services ample opportunity to do everything they could to prove they could understand my illness, and they had both failed, and destroyed my life, she/ he came right out with it and firmly stated that NOBODY was EVER going to look any further for a medical reason for my illness. There was not the slightest conception than any disease could escape detection after a few simple tests, and the words were said with no compassion or sympathy. Nails in my coffin were thudding home.

And things are worse than that: although this new clinic is actually in my own conurbation, the reason I was turned down was because I am still bureaucratically in a different CCG area, just as, previously, I had been in the wrong PCT area, and, just as happened three and a half years ago, I have not been referred out of area (with a six month wait, and pointless blood samples before being told this). The fact that this failure of referral involves exactly the same therapist, who I wasn't allowed to see the last time, is particularly ironic. And the local shrinks are still saying that 'I' have not 'co-operated' in obtaining treatment!

Worse still, this new CBT 'service', is ONLY for people who are not very ill. There will be no home visits or phone consultations for the really chronically ill. CBT is only for those with the good health and mobility to visit the shrines of the venerated doctors and shrinks, just like in the rest of the NHS. Psychiatry has infected the whole system to its very core. CBT is a 'success' because only those who don't need treatment are selected for it: for the rest of the 'Medically Unexplained Symptoms' spectrum, there is now, officially, NOTHING. For those in the very most need, it is the unashamed and official policy that they are left at home to suffer until they die.

We are, officially, the living dead.

We are despised: non-persons.

It is a crime against society to try to help us.

From Steve H

To the powers that be,

This letter is to all those people in authority who have disbelieved my children's invisible illness, pain and suffering over the past three years.

We are as you may know - but have questioned - a kind and caring family in which three out of four of us have ME, and the fourth has had his life wrecked unalterably by this illness. Our children were only seven and eleven when the disease took hold in a serious and life changing way for both of them and me as their mother.

From the start, those of you in education refused to believe that ME was incapacitating our children in the way it really was. You questioned the diagnosis, verified by two consultants specialising in ME. You told me one of my children had cancer, not ME. You refused to accept from these same consultants that my child needed to rest and be educated at home and told me instead she had to still come into school. You did not believe me when I said she was like the victim of a car crash.

Both you head-teachers of that era insisted my children looked well and made sure they were told this to their faces, so that they felt disbelieved and felt their illness was invalid. I am so angry still with you for this. You both refused to provide work so they could study at home, despite saying that you would. You covered up the abusive way some of your members of staff approached this illness. I know this so well as my friend's child with ME who had to still go to your school was marched around the playing field to wake her up! You told her to take a cold shower in the morning to be less tired. You refused her going home when she was sky high with fatigue. I feel so lucky my child was allowed medical tuition at home eventually and did not succumb to this torture.

You made me feel so bullied and afraid as a mum for standing up for them, especially as I myself have ME and could so easily by outsiders be perceived to be 'over-medicalising' my children's plight. I was told this only two weeks ago by my previously kind GP.

Eventually one of you made sure Social Services became involved and took this disbelief down the route of child protection.

This process was stopped dead in its tracks by the medics - but why did you do this to us a family? Why did you never try to support us all and allow us to speak up to your concerns? Everything was done behind our backs. Do you know what horrendous stress this caused and what shadows it continues to cast? We forever feel judged and observed, and every careful and thoughtful decision we make about treatment potentially scrutinised.

You will never know this, but the grief you have given us has been as immense at times as the heart-break ME has caused our family. You have not broken us, but you very nearly did.

We will never forget this. The scars of disbelief are there for the rest of our lives.

BUT we are, as you know, but refused to see, a kind and caring family who will always do the best for our children. We remain strong, not broken.

From a mum who does the best for her family. x

To my fellow teachers,

I'm going to ask you two things - please think about them as you read my letter:

What made you want to become a teacher?
Do you think that you are a good teacher?

There are so many different ideas about what makes a good teacher. As far the government is concerned, it's how many grades and levels you can churn out. To Ofsted it's how much progress kids make in a lesson. You can stay up all night and plan outstanding lessons, your kids can make more than three sub-levels of progress a year and don't get me wrong, it's important for them to learn, but in my mind just achieving that doesn't make you a good teacher. Ask any child and they won't say 'a good teacher allows me to make at least three sub-levels of progress a year'. You might get the odd few who say 'they let me sit there and do nothing, eat and get my phone out' (we've all had them, let's be honest) but the majority of kids will say that a good teacher listens, respects them, helps them solve problems and believes in them.

Which is why I can't quite agree with some teachers I've come across (and I stress the word 'some' - not all by a long way) who class themselves as good teachers.

In my current school, very few people know I have ME. That's just a personal choice which stems from a couple of things. One in particular is something I once heard which completely made me want to scream. I was talking to a teacher once on a course (not from my school) and somehow we got onto talking about ME. I hadn't told them that I had ME, but they were talking about a student who they taught who had it. This A grade student had gone from 100% attendance, perfect uniform, perfect behaviour to having three months off school after being diagnosed. As the girl's form tutor, this teacher had gone to a meeting the previous week to think about getting her back into lessons.

The teacher said to me 'but it's all just a load of rubbish isn't it? Maybe she's just trying to get attention because she's quiet or something... but she's no worse off than the rest of us. To be honest I think it's pushy parents looking for an excuse in case she doesn't get straight A's'.

Unfortunately, and I mean this out of no disrespect to my colleagues (especially as for a lot of them this completely does not apply) I have come across SO MANY attitudes like that, and sadly not just towards kids too, but to their colleagues at work. In my mind it goes completely against the idea of being a teacher - wanting to create good relationships with students and wanting to make a difference to them. How can you do either of those things when you're so quick to make a (very poor) judgement?

I know there are teachers who think that people with ME are just lazy whinge-bags who want to get the sympathy vote. Of course we all get tired, we all have to work hard, we all need the holidays (I've heard that one a few times). But as a teacher with ME myself, I know what it's like to be on the receiving end of those attitudes and it hurts. It makes you feel like you don't deserve to be human, that you are a total waste and it's pointless you doing the best you can because you'll never be good enough. Don't be fooled into thinking that this makes you want to give up though - in fact, you try to work even harder because you want to prove everyone wrong. You want to show that you are working just as hard as everyone else. But when you show that, you're met with 'see, they can do it, I knew it was an act' which just makes all the payback from your efforts that little bit more painful.

I tell you now that NOBODY would choose to live the life of an ME sufferer. As much as kids love being off school, that's maybe for a day - if they weren't genuinely ill surely they'd come back to be with their friends after a day or two because they were so bored and lonely? And who would seriously want doctors poking and prodding them relentlessly, being in and out of hospital? And can you SERIOUSLY imagine even the laziest student actually choosing to take such a significant chunk out of their own education? I know I can't think of any of mine who would purposefully miss out for so long, no matter how much they don't like school.

Those judgemental attitudes don't get to me as much anymore because I've learnt to not get so upset over them. But imagine what they do to a child? Imagine your whole life being taken away, your friends and the rest of the world moving on without you, and then being told that you are faking it or just lazy? And imagine how that would feel coming from someone you trust, see as a role model? Don't believe that not saying it to a sufferer's face doesn't mean they don't know how you feel. Unfortunately we are VERY sensitive to picking up on people's attitudes towards us. And to a child whose feelings and self-esteem may be lower anyway - well that could do some serious damage.

Students with ME need our love and care to help them succeed, just as any child does. They need us to be understanding when they choose to go to another lesson over ours, because too much will make them seriously ill again. They need our support in allowing them to complete assessments in small chunks rather than in one big go due to cognitive difficulties, so that they can feel at their best. They need our reassurance that we believe them and that we recognise that they are doing their absolute best. They need us to say to them 'I can see how hard you are trying and I appreciate it' rather than 'you managed to do that the other day, so you can do it today'.

Imagine that you came into work with full blown flu, right at the end of term, after having run a week-long residential trip in which you did a marathon every day. How would you want someone to respond to you?

So why did you decide to become a teacher, and a good one at that? If it was to judge your students and to brand them as lazy, refuse to understand why they can't just get on with it and refuse to change things just for them because you've got twenty-nine other kids to teach, then maybe you should look at a different career. But if it was to be that person who changed a child's life, and to be that person who was remembered in years to come for making a difference, then just try to see life through the eyes of a child with ME.

Lots of love from a teacher with ME.

To The Exams Officer at Secondary School,

Do you remember me? I remember you, the way you treated me will mean I can never forget you. The way you behaved might not have seemed harsh at all but that is where you are wrong.

I fell ill just as I entered Year 11 at school, GCSE year; the year that I had been told would determine how far I would get in life. My poor health meant that I wasn't able to come in to school anymore; I tried, I really did, and when I couldn't keep going I started having lessons at home. I was desperate to do my exams, but to you I was just another child trying to get out of coming to school.

I asked to have my exams in a quiet room, with breaks, snacks, drinks and extra time all of which you agreed to, or at least that's what you told us. When I arrived, when I was with other students, you banned me from eating and drinking and I wasn't able to take my breaks. What you didn't see is that when I got home I was exhausted and in agony both physically and mentally. I knew I couldn't keep going like this or I would fail all of my exams. This is where you got nasty. My poor mum fought for me, she fought so hard so that I could take the rest of my exams at home and all that time you put obstacles in our way.

When I came into school for my year photo didn't you see the wheelchair? Didn't you see the circles under my eyes? Didn't you see me trying so hard to sit up? Didn't you see me overwhelmed by the noise? You mustn't have done; someone who had seen that wouldn't have come up to my mum and say whilst tapping their watch 'I've noted that Sam was here today'. You were determined to make my life difficult.

The thing is, if you had taken that little bit of time to look at my school reports you would have seen that I was high achieving. If you had spoken to my teachers you would have heard that I tried my hardest in my classes. You'd have known that I wasn't perfect but I did my homework, I did my exams, I did after school clubs, I was in many school plays. Are these things that someone bunking off would do? Did the letters from specialists and GPs mean nothing to you? What gave you the right to think that you knew better than us?

But do you know what? I may have only got one B and two D's in my GCSEs, but that hasn't stopped me! I have a Level 3 Certificate which I'm aiming to turn in to a Diploma next year, I've done courses online. All of these things mean that I do have a future, but it also means I can support other young people who are in the situation I was in. I can be a role model and show them that there is a light at the end of the tunnel.

A Student Who Beat The Odds.

To my college,

I really enjoyed my time at college, but I wish you hadn't made things so difficult at the outset. When I was thinking of starting A Levels with you I had an interview. I told you that I had ME. I was realistic about what I would be able to cope with and told you everything I would need. You said all the right things. You promised me everything I said needed and even more. I was so excited to start college because I thought you were going to be so supportive.

I arranged with you to study one subject to start with, and that I would only be well enough to come in for one and a half lessons out of three a week. I was in for all the lessons I said I would be. I had no time off sick and always handed in my homework on time. I was so pleased when I was able to build up the length of time I was in lessons for faster than I had expected.

Imagine how shocked I was when you called me in to a surprise meeting and told me I wasn't doing enough. You got me on my own without my parents and told me I had to do more. I was so confused and upset. I was doing more than we had agreed, so why was it not enough? You pressured me and I felt bullied. I nearly cried. I knew if I agreed to do more that I would make my ME relapse. You placed me in an awful position. I could make you happy but in the process make myself ill, or continue doing what was best for me and make you angry or even risk being kicked out of college. I was doing everything I could and thought I was a model student. I always tried my hardest and did my best, so why did you make me feel like I was a skiver?

The turning point was one lesson. I had finished a project and only had to fill in a simple form in order to submit it, but it was the end of the lesson and I was exhausted. I had difficulty concentrating enough just to be able to fill in my name. No matter how hard I tried I could not fill in the rest of it. My mind felt like cotton wool and I couldn't string a sentence together. I just had one last box to fill in to explain what my project was about, but I had to tell my teacher I couldn't do it. She sat with me and told me word by word what to write and had to spell some of the words for me. She had finally seen what my ME could do to me. She finally understood what I was like when the lessons had finished and I went home. We'd told you I looked well in college and that my energy crashed when I got home, but I don't think you believed me until then. Finally you stopped pressuring me and I could get on with my studies.

In my second year, a girl in my class came down with glandular fever. I was shocked when I saw how supportive you were and how much you put yourselves out. You gave her everything you'd promised me in my interview but never actually delivered. You had told me you could send work home and that I could even do the whole course from home if I needed to, but when I asked you to send me work home you said it wasn't possible because of the nature of the course. I was annoyed at the time but when I saw you sending work home to my classmate it made me angry. Why did you go back on your promises to me? Why did you agree to do all these things and then never do them for me, while at the same time doing them all for someone else?

A few of your staff members were supportive. The lady who arranged all my exam concessions was wonderful. My teacher was finally supportive when she believed I was ill. All I ask is that in future you listen to people and don't go back on your promises. I was open and honest with you. I was realistic about what I could do and what I would need. I did everything that I said I would. I shouldn't have had to work so hard to prove myself to you. I think you were trying to make me better by pressurising me to do more, but I was already stretched to breaking point and you very nearly broke me. I came to do my A Levels with you because of the promises you made. The fact you didn't keep them could have been catastrophic. I had to rely on the friends I made in class to get the notes I needed for missing lessons. I couldn't have passed my first year without them. In the end I studied one A Level and one AS Level with you and got an A for both of them, but I feel that was because of my determination rather than the support I got from you. I hope that in future you will be more supportive of students with ME. Just because we don't necessarily look ill in lessons it doesn't mean we're putting it on. I saved up my energy for college so you saw me at my best. Next time, please listen.

Your ex-student.

I was seven and in Year 3

To my PE teacher,

    I felt ill, you didn't believe me. You shouted at me, you said 'this can't carry on'. I was shaking, tears were in my eyes. My parents had written a note, you didn't believe it but you didn't speak to them, you shouted at me and made me feel scared. I didn't understand what the problem was with you. I was scared when I walked past you in the corridor and it made me feel cold and shaky. I was so pleased when you stopped working at my school.

I am now eight and in Year 4

To my class teacher,

    I am still poorly but I feel safe. You understand me and look after me. I don't feel threatened any more. I am happy to come to school, even when I feel ill as I know you will take good care of me.

From Isla, aged eight

To Anna, my PGCE mentor,

What did you think when I first came to you in 2009? Was it along the lines of 'oh, she has ME, she's one of those'? Tell me honestly; did you pre-judge me?

When I first began my placement, I was doing really well. You said that I was well ahead of where you would expect me to be. The vibe that you'd given off before that I wasn't very good (although you probably never realised that you were doing it) faded and it was like you started to take me seriously. We'd even have a chat and a little laugh now and then! It felt like I'd finally got you on side and I'd also got the ME under control.

The thing with ME is that you can't sustain things like the amount of sheer graft I was putting into my teaching. That's not because you don't want to or you can't be bothered, and when I got to that stage it was like you turned on me. Suddenly, all the little jokes stopped and you were really off with me instead of stepping into my shoes. You didn't want to listen to me or understand me. You didn't listen when I told you how much I was trying, did you?

I spoke to my university tutor, not to complain about you but to ask for advice. She got in touch with you and explained that I'd been struggling. The nature of my illness meant that I needed a bit more support in managing my workload and pacing my classroom activities.

For a while you were really nice. It was like I'd got you on side again. But gradually, you became cold towards me again, despite my university tutors pointing out to you everything that I was doing well. You were even kind enough to tell me that if it was just up to you, you would have failed my placement because I didn't deserve to pass. You had no idea how much effort I was putting in, so that made me feel so angry.

You are incredibly lucky because you have your health. I don't, and that has a huge impact on my ability to do my job, and I really hope that you never have to experience what that is like because it is hell. You once said that ME is psychological because stress made it worse. But there are a lot of physical conditions that get worse with stress, and that doesn't make them psychological. Couldn't you see those physical symptoms or did you just choose to ignore them? I just wanted you to understand this:

ME IS A PHYSICAL ILLNESS. ME HAS PHYSICAL SYMPTOMS. IT IS NOT PSYCHOLOGICAL.

In the end, my university removed me from your school and sent me somewhere else. At that school, the first thing that my mentor did was sit down and listen to me explain what my condition was like, where I had problems and how we could work around them. I was allowed to stay at my new school for the rest of the year but by then the damage had been done; I'd made myself too sick and never managed to get back to my true ability as a teacher. I scraped through my PGCE, but everyone at that school understood and was supportive. I got a job there and my mentor was also my NQT mentor. I'm still there - this is my fourth year now. I've been part-time since my PGCE because I know that full-time is too much, but I'm managing, I'm surviving. I don't know if I'll teach forever, but I'm proud to have got this far.

You've probably mentored two or three more student teachers by now. They've probably been healthy and your life has been a lot easier.

I guess you weren't bad as a mentor to a healthy person, but I've just got a couple of pieces of advice for you. If you ever get someone with ME again, please, listen to them. Please try and understand them. Because whilst the illness is completely invisible to you, to them it is very real and you won't see them when they've gone home, when they are really ill and badly suffering, especially every single evening and weekend. Please understand that the holidays won't cure them, because unfortunately payback is not solved by just resting. And most importantly, just respect them for what they do and go through on a day-to-day basis. Because you seemed to only judge what you saw on the surface; next time, look a little bit deeper and I think you'll be surprised at just how much it takes someone to teach with ME.

From your old mentee x

To my ex-line manager,

I doubt you'll ever read this, and if you do, I doubt you'll know that this is to you. But I need to write it, because other people shouldn't have to put up with the rudeness and ignorance from you that I did.

I started my new job fresh-faced, eager, keen and excited. You were responsible for keeping an eye on my work and signing off my probation period. I'm sure (I'd hope) that it was nothing personal, but come the end of that period your manner left my confidence in bits.

Firstly, I'm going to tell you about when I left my job. I'd spent the month after my probation finished on sick leave (little did I know that I'd never go back) because of a different medical problem - I had a collapsed lung which needed surgery to repair. I emailed you, explained that I had decided to hand in my notice and spend that month-long period on sick leave (that wasn't so much a choice), thanked you for all you had done, because I felt that it was the right thing to do. I meant it, of course. But your reply that you were sorry that I'd been so ill, instead of making me feel better or cheered up, made me feel angry. You were *sorry*? So now that I had something that was clearly visible, and more accepted, you were sorry? It angered me because you had spent the whole of my probation period being completely stand-offish and actually quite rude when I was struggling. At times you questioned my professionalism. Actually, the way that you were towards me when I was having difficulty, THAT was unprofessional. And you had the nerve to be sorry when there was something that you could actually see?

You made it very clear, maybe not right from the start but certainly once you'd realised that I had ME, that you didn't like me. That wasn't a problem, I didn't care about that, but what I did care about was how you felt that it was appropriate to make me out to be rubbish at my job, when you full well knew that I wasn't. Instead of helping me do my job, you felt it necessary to tell me that I didn't think the standard that I needed to achieve was the same as the standard I actually needed to achieve. How you, an outsider to the many years of my life with this illness, felt that you were able to measure how hard I was trying, how ill I was making myself just to get through that period, is beyond me.

When I was off ill, the majority of my other colleagues, including YOUR boss, asked me how I was, whether I was feeling better, whether I should actually be in the office at all. You were cold and said that I'd find it hard to get back on track with things now that I'd had a few days off. You questioned me, asked me how I could still be feeling ill when I'd had time off and had been resting.

At other times, you named colleagues who had children unwell in the night, had long drives, had families, but they still managed to cope. I never wanted (and still never do want) to use my illness as an excuse, but you really did belittle the amount I had been suffering. You never attempted to try to understand that, you were just focused on assuming that I should become totally immersed in my job, just like you. That I should almost forget my illness because then it couldn't affect me during the working day. For your sake, I really hope that you never get ME yourself.

I got through my probation with the help of other people and their backup. I'd met my targets more than some people who had been there for years. When I had to reflect on my performance at the end, rather than congratulate me like everyone else was, you were really stroppy towards me, like you were angry that I'd made it. I'd wanted to please you before, but I never felt the need to from then on.

I could go on and on about the things that you did to make me feel so awful. How, during an assessment of my work, you would stand there and just frown (don't think for a second that others didn't pick up on that too, by the way). How you would slate me during feedback, when others had said that I'd done a good job. You just made out all the time that I simply wasn't trying. I could go on about how every time I've seen you since I left you've blanked me. How that really hurt at first. But actually, it doesn't bother me. I'm doing well at my new job now, because I can manage it and people are less judgmental than you.

I hope you never get ME, because with an attitude like you displayed, you'll never cope.

I may see you again, I may not. But I'll be sure to tell you how well I'm doing now that I have people around me who support me!

From an old employee - who will always strive to be NOT like you!

Dear Family...

To my family and many now so distant friends...

Why have you deserted me?

I know it is because of my ME and not me as a person. For these reasons I detest ME. It has robbed me of my life force, and each day I feel as if I am only existing; days just pass in a blur. I have to learn to be patient, very patient, in the hope that lots of resting will give me an hour or two of fun, or maybe if I am really lucky, a trip out for a few hours.

I have had to learn to let go of my past life; it is as if it were a dream, was that really me? Did I used to train with fellow athletes, teach them to be faster, better, more powerful? Did I really have my own sports therapy clinic; did I really massage Girls Aloud? Was it me that competed in triathlons all around the country?

Who am I now? What do I like? I do not know, I just like to be happy - I cannot do much else.

I like to hear from people, to live my life through them, to hear about the fun, the adventures they had. I want to feel part of that in any way possible.

You have deserted me, my family, and now so distant friends; slowly you stopped trying.

I have one good friend left - she knew me at my fittest; she was the fittest female along with myself that I knew. She calls, she makes me giggle, she shares her life with me and understands our illness. For that reason she makes me cry too, for she knows the truth and what I want to still be and what I have become. She knows I have such a disabling illness and I thank her from the bottom of my heart for her understanding.

I hate the stigma behind ME; see my past - I am not lazy, I love exercise, I even tried damn Graded Exercise that would have been too easy for an old lady forty years my senior! You see, I did not want to give up, I wanted to get better; it made me worse, my ME does that. It is like a nasty life-sucking monster that sucks your energy and strength, and the more you fight it the worse you become. ME, you are like a black hole sucking us into your universe where no-one can see us, shut away. I have a voice though that cannot be silenced; whilst I am here I shall keep talking - for there are millions like me who detest, hate and would do anything to rid the world of ME.

All I ask is please believe in ME. I have come to know online my cyber friends who suffer from all walks of life. The most courageous, bravest, wonderful friends of all, fighting for our voices to be heard; it horrifies me to learn there were so many at first - the scale of the damage of ME is fast becoming a humanitarian crisis of neglect.

Xxxxx

To my family and friends, and to everyone,

Please, I really want all of you to understand that we don't choose to be ill; we want the normal pain-free lives that you all take for granted, the freedom you won't realise you have until you have lost it. The freedom from constant pain that we can only dream of - and the freedom from the 'fibro fog', confusion and the muddled sentences when we push ourselves too far.

Everything we do, every concentrating thought that we have can knock us literally from our feet at times. There is a piece of writing called 'The Straw Theory' that if all our families and friends could possibly take the time to read, and then if you could then take the time to talk to your family member or friend that has ME/ CFS and/ or Fibromyalgia, then we each of us would be more than happy to talk to you. We are not being lazy or exaggerating; any of the other misconceptions that you may have about what we have are wrong. We are just ill people trying to get better and to live our lives. No-one would choose to have this, but we need people to start listening and talking to educate each other, and especially to understand.

Love, H.

To my brother,

I feel so lucky to have you as my brother. I know that a lot of things have changed because of me being ill. It was a while before I realised that my illness had completely changed life for you too. We went from doing things like horse-riding and tennis lessons to suddenly not being able to do any of those things, or go out as a family. There were so many fun things we used to do that we couldn't anymore. In a way, I'm surprised you didn't resent me more because of it. Yet in many ways you've made my ME much easier. For example, I remember the first time I had to use a wheelchair I was really self-conscious and hated the fact I had to use one. You made it fun and I really enjoyed it. After that, we went out and bought a wheelchair, and could start going out as a family again. Coming to terms with using a wheelchair was one of the best things I did and you made it so much easier.

I'm sorry that sometimes my ME has made me grumpy. You must have thought I had awful mood swings and could be a stroppy cow sometimes! I'm not as bad as I used to be, but sometimes when I feel exhausted I just don't have the energy to cope with things. It means when you tease me I find it funny when I'm feeling well, but need to be left alone when I'm feeling ill. I don't ever mean to snap at you and I've felt guilty whenever I have done, but sometimes I just can't help it because I feel really awful and just need to be left alone. I don't always have the energy to explain how I'm feeling or what I need.

Sometimes it has been hard having you around whilst I've been ill. It's like I have a well person to compare myself with and I can see all the things I might have done. I would have loved to be well enough to go to university. You went to Cambridge, one of the best universities in the world, and I was never well enough to go away to any university at all.

When you came home from university for the holidays I loved having you around, but sometimes it was hard because it reminded me of what I was missing. I had fun hanging out with you and my friends, but when I had to go home early because I wasn't well enough to stay out longer, but you could stay out for as long as you liked, I found it very upsetting. It was depressing lying in bed and hearing you come in at 2am knowing you'd been out having fun with my friends. You could do things with my friends that I never could.

I love having you as my brother. Thank you for putting up with me and being so supportive of my ME. It's meant I've always had one friend my own age who has been understanding. Thank you for all the things you've done for me like coaching me for my Physics GCSE and picking me up from college. I couldn't ask for a better brother.

With love,

Your sister xxxxx

Dear Dad,

Do you think this is how I want to live my teenage years? That I choose to be ill all this time, that I choose to not be able to spend time with my family and friends?

You make me feel like my illness is a huge burden to you. You make me feel so embarrassed about needing a wheelchair when in reality it's not an embarrassment - I need to be able to go out and without it I wouldn't have gotten out of my house for years. Why is it so hard for you to just smile, to make me feel okay to go out in my wheelchair with you, to make me feel comfortable?

I know I haven't stayed at your house for a few years now but I really want to! I can't stay for a number of reasons; you don't have a downstairs toilet so I can't get up and down the stairs eight to ten times a day because of my over active bladder (an ME symptom). I go to bed at 10pm every night and wake up at 8am every morning due to my pacing which is how I'm getting better. So I can't stay, because that would mean you all doing the same - because I have to sleep downstairs, due to there being no room upstairs for me to sleep!

When you say things like 'I just feel sorry for you because you're missing out on the best years of your life', that doesn't help. That makes me feel ten times worse because I already know that. I'm missing out on normal teenage years - I can't go out with my friends, go shopping, go on long nights out or even drink alcohol.

I know it must be hard looking in and seeing my life and how normal I look and act when I'm around you, but that's not how I am when I get home. When I get home I go to bed and sleep for hours on end. Please, just before you say things or do things, think how hard it is for me, how difficult every day is. Then you might choose to phrase things differently or to not say them at all.

Love, ME, your daughter

Dear Mum,

Look Mum!

Look Mum I'm growing in you
Look Mum see me grow?
Look Mum do you love me?
Look Mum I've arrived
Mum, Mum, can you see ME?

Look Mum I'm smiling
Look Mum I'm crawling
Look Mum I'm walking
Look Mum I'm talking
Mum, Mum, can you see ME?

Look Mum I'm good
Look Mum I will be quiet
Look Mum I can write my name
Look Mum I will be a big girl
Mum, Mum, can you see ME?

Look Mum I am sick
Look Mum I am hiding
Look Mum I am loving you
Look Mum I don't like Dad
Mum, Mum, can you see ME?

Look Mum I am reaching out to you
Look Mum I am loving you
Look Mum I forgive you
Look Mum you can't love ME.

To my mum,

In the beginning, the symptoms of ME soared and overtook me at a great rate. As I spun trying to take it all in and understand it before diagnosis, I also spun for real, overcome with vertigo. Thankfully you were there to witness my struggle, to care for me and my children as I retreated to my room and to my bed. As a Christian I cried out to the Lord 'what is going on? Please bring me comfort. How I wish you were here with me now, to hold my hand and stroke my head!' Moments later you entered my room and sat on my bed. You held my hand. You leaned over and stroked my head. Even though you might not share some of my beliefs, you were the hands and feet of Jesus to me in a time of deep need. You showed me the one thing that would transcend all else. Love.

You have been such an integral part of my journey Mum, and your support and love has helped me through many times.

Thank you <3

Dear Mum,

I don't blame you for not understanding me. I don't blame you for wanting me to try harder, to just get on with life. I don't blame you for questioning me when I have a bad day, because I know that this illness is invisible and you can't see the pain I'm going through. But I do want you to know just how difficult your lack of understanding makes it for me.

When they suspected that I had ME, you told me not to get a diagnosis because I would never get a job. At the time I was really angry but now I can see that you were just voicing your concerns about my future. In fact, I can see now that a lot of the times that I thought you were just being cruel were just because you didn't want me to fail in life. I promise that it was never my intention to fail, and I haven't failed at all; it's just that not all my achievements are achievements in your mind.

Shortly after being diagnosed, I spent months bed-bound, living a very miserable and lonely life because I'd pushed too hard. And at that time I needed your understanding and your support so much. I know you thought that you did understand and that you were supporting me, but it felt like if I couldn't do something, or wanted to take things at my own pace, in your eyes I was putting barriers up and I didn't really want to get better. You didn't just hurt me emotionally but also physically too; I wanted you to accept that I really was trying to get better and so pushed and pushed, and it just made the payback so much worse. I hated that you'd refuse to have my wheelchair in the house or that you made such a big thing of me needing carers. I wanted you to see that I hated it too, but I needed you to reassure me that it was OK. I wanted you to accept my situation for what it was, and believe that I was still the same person.

Eventually I came through it, moved away and managed to get myself a full-time job. It felt so good to feel like you accepted me again and that you were proud of me, so much so that I didn't want to tell you about how I was still suffering because I didn't want to break that pride. That's why I don't tell you things now, because I don't want you to get upset or feel like I'm not trying my best. Recently deciding to leave my job that I loved so much was the hardest decision in the world for me, and I know to you it must have looked like I was just giving up. But you could never understand why I did it. Every night I was coming home too exhausted to function and it was so painful; I was making myself very ill. I didn't expect you to understand what it felt like when I tried to tell you at all, but I just wanted you to believe me instead of telling me that you got tired too but still managed.

I find myself now in a situation where I will be successful, but maybe not in the way you'd planned. I hope that you can accept that but I want you to understand the reasons behind it too. This illness is so bewildering for me even after so many years of living with it so I need to know that you will listen, believe and reassure me when I struggle. I need you to accept my limitations instead of me having to push and suffer just because I'm so scared of making you angry. I need to know that I can tell you things, not keep them from you just so that you'll stay proud of me. Because I hate keeping things from you. I want to make you proud not by achieving high promotions or earning an amazing salary, but just by going through what I go through on a daily basis and refusing to give up.

Because at the end of the day, I may well have this illness for the rest of my life, but that doesn't change who I am.

Xx

To my mum,

>Thank you for believing in me.

When I hear the words 'believing in me', it makes me think of believing that someone is strong enough to do something. That they have what it takes to do what they have to do.

Maybe sometimes it even means believing them, that they are telling the truth. That they really are suffering. That they are not just making things up.

You have done both of these things for me. But even more you have just simply believed in me. You believed I still existed when I thought not. You still saw me as a mother when I could not. You still saw the artist in me when I did not. You still saw the fighter in me when I gave up. You still saw me within the frame of ME, and in time I saw me too and started to believe. For that I will always be grateful. There is no greater gift you could give me than to have never given up or lost sight of who I really am.

I love you mum xo

To my parents,

> How could you?

I don't know if you will ever read this but I want you to know how I feel.

You have never believed or accepted my illness.

In the early days you told me to pull myself together and get back to work.

You have said that it's all in my mind.

You have said that I am lazy.

How can you not know your own daughter?

How could you have talked to me like that?

How could you abandon your own daughter?

How could you refuse to speak to your own daughter?

How could you say that she no longer existed?

How could you stop sending her birthday cards as if she no longer existed?

How could you not even be concerned and ask about me when I went into hospital?

How could you look right past me as if I'm not there?

How could you walk past me in the street and ignore me as if I'm a ghost?

How could you talk to others about me and say cruel and hurtful things?

All I wanted was your help and support.

All I wanted was to know that you cared.

All I wanted was your acceptance that I was ill.

All I wanted was your acknowledgement that I was your daughter.

All I wanted was your love.

I have felt abandoned, neglected, hurt and lonely.

What have I ever done to deserve this sort of treatment?

I thought a parent's love was unconditional.

I hope that one day the truth will come out and you will have cause to be sorry and ashamed for how you have treated your own daughter.

xx

To my parents,

Thank you for everything you have done for me. I don't think I would have been able to cope with having ME if it weren't for you.

You did all the research about ME when I was too ill to do it myself. To be honest, I was so young and emotionally shaken up about being ill that I don't think I could have managed to research it even if I'd had the energy.

You've cooked, cleaned, done my washing and all the other things I've needed you to do over the years. I really appreciate that when I have energy you let me do some fun things like going out with you or spending time with friends, rather than letting me spend all my energy on looking after myself and just existing. You've made sure I've had some fun even though I've been ill.

You've let me focus my energy on the things I want to do. I couldn't possibly have managed to get any GCSEs and A Levels or currently be working towards a degree if it weren't for you. Everything I have achieved, you have made possible.

You've driven me around to doctor's appointments, alternative therapy sessions, school lessons, college lectures and to see my friends. I would have been totally housebound for years if you hadn't been willing to take me everywhere I wanted to go and pick me up again. You let me have my friends over when I wasn't well enough to go out and even tidied up afterwards for me. You did everything you could to make sure I had some social life.

You protected me from the pediatrician who gave me the wrong advice and made me worse. You dealt with my school when they were unhelpful. You coped with all the stress so I didn't have to. You supported me when my home tutor was difficult. You didn't let my college bully me. You were there when my friends weren't. You've helped me work out my pacing plan and stick to it so now I'm getting better. Most importantly you believed me when I said I was ill.

You have done everything a parent could to support and care for their child. I know my ME has greatly affected our family. It's made daily life much more difficult and stressful. It's stopped us from doing many things like days out and going away on holiday. You've always taken care of me and you've never ever complained. There is no way that I can ever thank you enough for what you have done and still continue to do.

Xxx

Open letter from a mother caring for two daughters with ME;

Sometimes I want to scream and shout at the universe, WHY? Why my children?

I am the mother and full-time carer of two daughters with ME. My youngest daughter was ten years old and just starting Year 6 of primary school when she fell foul of the illness, resulting in her leaving school by the November of the first term and has not been able to return since. She is now fourteen and only just become well enough to manage an hour of home tuition twice a week. My other daughter with ME became sick when she was fourteen; she had viral meningitis and never seemed to recover and developed ME on the back of that - she is now almost sixteen, out of education and trying hard to manage fifteen minutes of home tuition twice a week.

Life, it has to be said, can be exceptionally unfair. Caring and loving for our chronically ill children is tough - not the physical doing of, but the having to watch them going through the many bad days which are full of pain, anxiety, fatigue and frustration, yet being absolutely helpless in the ability to ease their suffering. All I can do is let them know I am there, loving and supporting them as best I can whilst acknowledging their distress.

There are times when trying to give basic motherly love is impossible - when just holding them close hurts their skin, the light hurts their eyes, food brings on extreme nausea and the slightest noise makes their head ring. It has been known for me to not use the hoover for weeks at a time because they can't bear the noise it makes.

Yet, through all this I am astounded at their tenacity and humour, their ability to make the best of the hand life has dealt them. They are a constant source of pride and inspiration; I find it is incredible how strong they are and the depth of maturity for their age, and most of all the desire to still help others whilst suffering themselves.

As a child you just take for granted the fact that you can go to school, gain an education, go out and get up to mischief with your friends and just live life to the maximum without any worries - it's just what you do, isn't it?

For our family and sadly many others I have since been in contact with, with children suffering from ME, this isn't so.

The girls have sorely missed the day-to-day routine of school life and friendships that you would normally take for granted. We wasted years trying to send them into school on a seriously reduced timetable which didn't work, and then going to a school room in the Children's Hospital for just a few hours a week, which again didn't work due to the brain fog and physical symptoms of the illness, which left us floundering and the girls at home with no education. Now they have small pockets of home tuition but it isn't really enough for them to gain any qualifications - we are resigned to them having to pursue them later in life via adult education.

Another big issue for the girls is depression, anxiety and panic attacks, which are crippling at times and can be so severe they cause full blackouts. We understand why they suffer like this - they are grieving for a childhood and friendships lost, and suffer from anxiety due to becoming more and more isolated and housebound.

Both girls suffer cruelly and we have to utilise the wheelchair and/ or crutches to go out. We have a shower stool so that they can bathe (as baths are too difficult for them to get in and out of, depletes their energy too severely) and on bad days we have to resort to wet wipes, dry shampoo and chewable toothbrushes. They also suffer from hypermobility, IBS and POTS - quite common, I have since found out, for people with ME to suffer with these alongside the illness.

We live our days in a bubble - these four walls have become our world. We venture out rarely, but when we do we try to make the absolute best of it and squeeze out each moment of pleasure we can. We have lost contact with many members of our family and most of our friends - they just don't, or won't, understand the illness and the impact upon our lives, despite us sharing information with them about it.

I am hoping that there will be a day in the future - not too far away, when the health professionals will accept that this is a very real, cruel, debilitating physical illness and NOT psychological. I am praying for treatments to become available, awareness and understanding by the general public and that sufferers aren't left ostracised and left to their own devices, struggling to cope as best as they can any more.

Yours in hope, a desperately sad mother.

To my children,

>I want you to know that I love you.

When I'm having a bad day laid out on the couch and you come and ask me to play, and I say 'not today'. Know that I love you.

When I'm in bed and you come and ask me to make you some breakfast, and I say 'just watch one more cartoon, and then I'll get up'. Know that I love you.

When I am not there to pick you up from school and you have to have someone else take you home again. Know that I love you.

When I fall asleep half-way through the movie that you really wanted me to watch. Know that I love you.

When I'm resting in my hammock outside and you ask me to come and play in the pool with you, and I say 'Mummy needs rest'. Know that I love you.

When you ask me to read to you and I say 'I have a headache today, why don't you read it to me?' Know that I love you.

I love you, my children, with all of my heart and I am doing my best. Your childhood is short and precious - you are growing so fast. You are becoming such wonderful people. I am proud of you, my charismatic young man and my sweet princess.

Mummy has ME. That means Mummy's body is sick and Mummy needs lots of rest. My body doesn't make enough energy to play. But my heart works perfectly, and it is full of love for you.

Don't hold yourself back because of me, play and laugh with each other. I hope you live vibrant lives full of colour and love.

I hope against hope that this family curse ends with me. But know if you ever do find yourself ill I will look after you. Together we will build the best life we can. Together we will be OK.

Love from Mummy.

To my three beautiful sons,

Where would I be without you three? Without all the love and acceptance you have shown me? I was so taken aback to find that when I was able to do nothing for you because I had ME, you still loved me and loved to be near me. Even at the ages of one, five and nine you brought so much support into my world with your hugs and smiles. No adult can match what you have given me.

You would search me out when I was encaved by my bed, bringing me gifts of love in hugs, kisses, drawings, playing with your toys beside me or curling up in my cave with me for a sleep together. You filled the spaces on the couch beside me when all I could do was sleep and watch TV (and still do now at ages nine, thirteen and seventeen). You showed me the true meaning of love. That it can't be earned. You showed me my value in just being me, and in simply being your mum. You showed me the true meaning of family, being together and accepting each other.

Thank you, my three beautiful sons, for simply being yourselves and bringing so much comfort, love, hope and joy into my ME world. May each of you be blessed throughout your life with the same love you have shown me.

Love your mum xo

To my darling Erin,

On this day, as I write this, you have turned twenty-six months old.

These have been the most precious twenty-six months of my life and they will grow with every second, minute, hour, day, week, month and year I spend with you, my beautiful daughter.

Everyone always talks about that special bond between a mother and child, but never will you begin to appreciate it, and not take it for granted, until you are a mother yourself. One day, I will have to explain to you why Mummy can't do things with you that other mums do with their children, why I am nearly always tired and/ or in pain. Maybe you will be jealous of other children. Maybe you will be angry and upset with me for not being the parent you feel you deserve, but maybe, just maybe, one day, you will understand.

I have been unwell with ME for many years. It's hard to tell how many. I was diagnosed in 2007, but it is suspected I have had some form of the illness since 1993. For those first fourteen years, I worked hard, tried hard and cried hard when it all got too much, thinking that I shouldn't be struggling. Not understanding why I had to put in so much more than others in order to get the same result.

Getting a diagnosis was a relief, though scary and confusing. I was terrified that I would be alone forever and that I wouldn't be able to have the one thing I wanted more than anyone else in the world. How ironic then, that only three or so months after my diagnosis, I met your dad and sister and here we are today.

Throughout our time together, I couldn't have hoped for a better daughter. If we get on as well when you are older as I feel we do now, I will never need to worry.

Since having you, although there have been hard times with my feeling ill, no day has ever felt totally unbearable. You make me smile when I think no-one else can. You've pretty much slept well, though as I write this, you are sleeping fitfully because you are teething. You seem to accept my limitations as the norm now. It scares me that this will likely change in the not too distant future.

Please know that I will always be here for you, I will always do everything I can for you without question, and my love for you cannot be rivalled. You are everything to me, you have changed my life for the better, and for that I cannot describe my pride in you, my thanks, or my admiration for someone who is still so small.

All my love forever and always, Mummy

Dear Leah,

Now that you're at the age to understand a bit more about my illness, it is a relief in a way to be able to talk to you a bit about it and explain why I can't do as much as other people. At the same time though, it really does worry me how much you seem to worry and almost obsess about how, because bad things happen to other people, that means that they will happen to you. That's not the way the world works sweetheart, and I tell you this with an ache in my heart because I wish I could make you appreciate and understand that right now, so that you do not spend any more time agonising about such things. I used to be just like you in that way, in so many ways in fact. You are far too young to be worrying about the things that you do. You need to enjoy life, especially your childhood, as much as you can. You will have plenty to worry about later on in life.

I've recently found a book, aimed at children, which tries to explain ME a bit more. I am going to buy it for you. I just hope that it isn't too much for you to take on and try to understand.

Unfortunately for you, in the past, and still now to a degree, you seem to get the brunt of my temper if I am in a bad mood when you are here. I can never express how sorry I am for that. I try so hard not to snap at you. I think it is getting better, but that is no excuse. I get very tired very easily, and I have a lot of pain in my body, and when that happens, I just want to shut myself away. Your sister will grow up knowing no different to a degree, so it will maybe be easier with her, but you're not here often enough to appreciate that it's not like that all of the time, and it's definitely not you or anything you've done.

If I am honest, I feel like I always have to match up to some kind of expectation. You do different things when you're at your mum's. Maybe more, but maybe just different, and I always feel like I have to compete with that somehow. Not because I want to, but because I want to do enough to make sure that you're not bored, or that you don't decide that you want to go home early. He never says much, but I know it breaks your dad's heart to see you leave early because it's not exciting enough for you here. Why shouldn't you feel like that? You're just a child, but unfortunately adults see things in different ways.

I love you very much, but the one thing that I want to tell you is that it is exhausting being a stepmother with ME. I know you say it's OK that I snap, and I really hope you mean that, but it isn't. I just hope as you grow up you will understand where I'm coming from a bit more. I love having you here, spending time with you and doing as much as I can with you. Never doubt it.

Love Danielle

To my husband,

    Why do you blame me, give me the cold shoulder and make me feel so lonely? It's not my fault I struggle to balance married life, a young child, looking after a house and unpacking, and trying to get a job to help us get out of debt.

I may look better to you than this time last year, but you don't see my tablet box or know what I take when; you don't see me in pain in bed at night because you're too busy refusing to grow up, playing computer games or having a social life.

All I'm asking for is a little help around the house to keep it clean, and with looking after our son. When he's been really poorly for days, who is the one up all hours comforting and dealing with him whilst feeling rubbish myself?!

You don't realise how good you've had it or have got it now! I get up early so you can sleep, never getting a lie in because even when your parents have our son my body clock gets me up. You get up pretty much before you have to leave for work. When not volunteering or having interviews I'm trying to keep the house tidy, putting dishes away, getting washing done etc. after the morning school run. I then do the afternoon school run and make sure there is a hot, cooked meal on the table for when you get home. You then go straight on the computer once you've said goodnight to your son, after I've gotten him ready and read him a story, and I go and lie in bed watching a few episodes from a series before trying to sleep so that I can get out of bed when our son wakes.

At the weekend, you sleep until lunch if not longer, leaving me to deal with the bad behaviour as our boy can't cope without the structure of school. And also, why the hell can't you accept that he probably has ADHD and do things the same way as me and the school? It would make things easier on all of us if we worked off the same page.

I know you love me, otherwise you would have left last year when divorce was mentioned, when we went through the bad patch - when I struggled even more as I was so poorly.... how I stayed out of bed/ hospital I do not know.

I just would like to feel more appreciated and supported.

This illness takes so much away without you making me sacrifice so much on top, so that our son grows up happy and in a nice house with home-cooked food. I have made a few good friends at school gates but hate not being able to have a social life as I feel too tired or poorly to do anything. And the times I rarely have fun I then feel judged by you.

I love you and always will. You are my friend, my soul mate and my husband and I can't imagine life without you, but I just wish you could see it from my perspective or live some time in my shoes.

Your wife. x

To my husband,

The last eighteen months could have been the toughest of our twenty-five year marriage, but somehow we have become closer and our marriage has become stronger.

Your total support has been, and indeed still is, very much appreciated.

I guess we were lucky, because this illness didn't hit our lives until after our family was almost grown-up. We were fortunate to both have strong health for so long. I have amazing memories of our exploits walking, camping, swimming, cycling and so much more, both as a couple and with our children. We certainly lived life to the full.

I am grateful for all these times.

However, I appreciate that in changing my life, ME has also changed your life. And I love you all the more, for how you have helped me find new ways to enjoy life. The mobility scooter has been a life-saver for me. Your helping me buy a second-hand one so quickly after the idea was raised allowed me to cope with the transition to being 'disabled' more easily.

I love how you have found new ways for us to enjoy time together that don't involve physical challenges. Yet I am relieved that you still head out cycling with your friends and come back home with all the usual stories!

Accepting my new limitations has not been easy, but you have never doubted how much this illness affects me, nor tried to push onto me your own views about how I should cope with it. Some friends find this concept very difficult, because they see every problem as having a solution. You recognise that ME isn't that simple and that I need to find my own balance. That can't be easy when I make mistakes time and again!

I know we are both taking a 'one day at a time' approach, and neither of us has discussed the future much. For now I prefer this approach. I guess I'm still hoping that I'll just magically wake up cured one morning. Whatever way the future goes I am grateful for your patience with my new quirks. I hope I would have been as strong had our fates been reversed.

Really I don't think I'd have managed without your support and love. Thank you!

With love,

K.

PS - Oh and that new little routine of taking time for a kiss in the morning as you head out to work - I especially love that! x

To my hubby,

> I know this hasn't been easy for you.

In many ways ME has attacked you at the core as aggressively as it has attacked my body. I know it's been hard for you to accept. I have seen you struggle as your dreams went down the drain, just as mine did. No wife for a playmate, to go out with, to dream with. All the things that we may have achieved together that would take physical strength, blown away in the wind. The financial burden of providing for your family falling squarely and only on your shoulders.

I have seen you grow through this experience into a more patient and tolerant person. I know that process has been painful, sometimes for both of us. I hope that with acceptance, new dreams can come forth for us to achieve together and our future again can be bright.

Love Ali xo

Dear husband,

I know you love me and are sympathetic to my illness, but could you actually try to really understand what I'm feeling?

I'm not feeling 'tired' or 'weary', I'm feeling totally wiped out and exhausted, and when I'm active it's hard work to ignore the pain. You don't need to remind me not to do too much.

I'm feeling angry that I'm like this, especially as you don't appreciate the good health you still have - and I always enjoyed mine. I'm feeling frustrated as I watch you sit around wasting your energy when I could be using it.

I'm feeling really sad that I've realised you actually prefer me like this because I'm now always at home instead of out having fun. I now rely on you and you like it.

I don't want to, but I couldn't do without you.

xxx

To my man,

A marriage not what we expected. Us both having ME we knew what this disease could do, but wedded bliss put that aside. Our tiny, illness-friendly wedding. Our comfy, happy life, despite malaise, fatigue, pain. Even those we shared. Feeling each other's symptoms, both knowing what it's like.

Then moderate ME became severe. The honeymoon years were replaced with ones of unhappiness, fear and tears. Glasses of wine and walks in the rain with spoon feeding and commodes.

You watched in terror during the times I shook uncontrollably, couldn't stop vomiting, fell unconscious... you held my hand, not knowing what to do, when I cried dawn 'til dusk, trembled in panic, begged for you to kill me. You turning away broken-hearted, not being able to ease my suffering, swap places, make me happy anymore.

I became horrible to you, you to me. I even feebly threw something at you once. ME brought out the worst in us. Traits neither knew were there.

You wanted to leave, to escape, yet you stayed. Joyless, lonely days for you. Days of a bachelor but with the responsibility of a wife barely alive. Existence and not much more.

Whilst you dealt with your own failing health I couldn't be there for you. When you returned from your mother's death bed to hold me up, I could do nothing for you. From one horror to another.

No romance, no fun, no laughing. I cannot care for you as a wife should, cannot cook your tea, sew on your buttons. So one-sided. You took on the world of cooking, household chores, cleaning the fish tank. You became a carer. Until your ME took over and you could do it no more.

I cannot understand fully what it was like for you, you cannot for me despite yourself once knowing the misery of being bedridden. But I do know they were the worst days of your life. And the worst days of mine.

Yet you stayed, and here you are still. Would another man have done this? Faithful, loyal, a Goliath in support. Telling me I was beautiful when I looked a haggard wreck. Always promising better days whilst I listened in disbelief. Rubbing cream on my feet. Silly songs, daft faces, trying to make me laugh. Unsuccessful but appreciated. Although maybe not at the time.

I am forever grateful. I could not ask for more. Your forgiveness, your devotion, your strength. 'We are a team', you say. A team that will win.

There are better days ahead for us; we shall be happy once again. We shall come out of this together having passed the test, refined and bonded stronger.

With love xxxxx

Dear You,

ME is a lonely illness. One which people don't understand. One which cuts you off from the outside world and limits your contact with people.

I wish I'd known about it much sooner, but it took years of struggling through life, causing relationship problems with family and friends - well they disappeared.

If only someone had understood. The problem was in my body, not my mind. I got depressed with the exhaustion, the pain, the muddled head, forgetfulness - so they said it was depression, and you believed them and still pushed me on beyond my physical limits, with threats if I didn't do what you wanted me to. So I tried.

I just got more and more sick. More and more isolated. More and more lonely.

The children grew up and moved on. That's what children do, and then they have children as well.

By then I was very sick, and finally after many years I was diagnosed with ME. I cried with relief that there was a name for what made me so sick, so exhausted, so much pain. Then I cried when they told me there was no cure, but still you didn't understand; still you wanted more, and then were the times you hurt me - physically. I couldn't fight back. I hadn't the strength.

There was only you and me left and you had a life to lead. Your work was your life. I was alone.

If only you had understood it could have helped me so much, but still after all those years no-one understood.

I wish the family kept in touch more. I know they're all busy but even a text message means so much. A visit means the world to me.

You finally retired. You're not the type to sit around and I'm not able to go out much, so you have filled your life with other things. I understand that you need people. You need to be part of the community. I understand that and just wish I was able to do the same.

Our grandchildren are growing up and I rarely see them. They too have busy lives. No time to visit, no time to talk, no time to email, no time to text.

Now I'm getting old. I've passed my 'threescore years and ten'. There have been other things wrong with my body. I didn't know they could all be connected. All auto-immune diseases. I found that out myself. No-one linked them.

I've found other people with the same illness. That has been such a relief. I have friends. People who understand, people who care. I feel for them. I feel so much for the young ones who are facing the unknown. I pray the researchers find the cause and then a cure whilst these young ones can still marry and have a family. They can have a proper life where fights for benefits, wheelchairs and other aids are no longer needed.

I am blessed that I know the joy of children and grandchildren. I just wish they remembered me more often.

I have done my best.

Love, Isobel

xxxxxx

Dear Janet and Julie,

You have no idea about the many ways in which you help me each and every day.

You make laugh when I'm down - clinical depression, sadness due to my situation, or during flare-ups.

You cuddle me through the pain - or should I say 'more pain than usual'.

You keep me amused through insomnia - which is ironically something I deal with a lot.

You soothe me when I'm angry - who wouldn't be angry from time to time in my shoes?

You sleep next to me during my daytime naps, letting me know that you're there, because when a wave of fatigue hits you sometimes all you can do is sleep it off.

You don't care what I look like - that I live in my PJs, that I haven't got the energy to brush my hair, or just look extra rubbish due to skin complaints or the latest bug I've caught thanks to my awful immune system.

You give me a reason to get out of bed in the morning... or afternoon... or evening - by looking after you, I look after myself.

You give me purpose in my small, insular world - something that is hard to come by when you're too sick & unreliable to work, too tired to create and don't want to bring anyone else into your exhausting life.

You make me smile, laugh and my heart sings every day with your love, your funny little idiosyncrasies and crazy antics.

You take me for who I am - no more, no less.

No questions, no 'how are you?'s, no explanations, no medical speak, no 'pep talks', no funny looks, no evil stares, no 'I know how you feel's, no exclamations that you look very well for someone so sick, no incredulity, no 'I get tired too's... just unconditional love and affection.

You may only be babycats but my life is a million times better with you in it. The sound and vibration of your purrs as you lie in my arms is the most healing thing I know. Your kitty kisses and head bumps say 'I love you' in a pure and unadulterated way.

In short you help me through hard times, share the good times and are there for all that's in between.

For this, and countless other things, I love and thank you with all my heart... I could do without the 4am serenading though.

xoxo

Dear Lord,

     I don't know why you made this choice for me. I know you are good – you've shown me you are in so many ways. And yet in this one way, understanding your goodness remains elusive to me, your meaning a mystery.

At the beginning there was much prayer, much hope, much believing for the miracle. When that didn't happen there was also much courage. I felt the anticipation of a battle well fought; the honour of valour in the face of adversity.

As the years have passed, I've worn the well-trod paths between anger, hope, desperation and determination, and I've survived. More than that, I've lived. A good life – a blessed life. And I've believed in you, loved you, and known you to be true. And yet my trust in your choices for me has eroded. Is it your wisdom I've doubted, or your love? Maybe your sovereignty, your power. I'm not sure.

I've tried to take control of my health, my body, my future, rather than trust them to you. And I've stopped talking to you about it, stopped asking, because the pain of another 'no' was too great. Inevitably our intimacy – the joy of our love – has grown cold. What is love without trust, without communication, without life together? It is a fact of a relationship, not a living one.

The years have left me tired now. So tired, so desperately tired. I'm tired of the daily, minute-by-minute struggle to make my body move, to function.

The struggle to make my tired brain think, process, plan, assess. The struggle to make my heart keep hoping, keep warm, keep loving, and keep trying.

The struggle for help, for recognition; fighting against the paralysing fear of doctors. Living with the terror of what my future may hold if I can't convince someone to help me.

The stress and strain of that terrible pressure of being responsible, in every decision I make, every action I take, for the consequences to my body, my husband, my family, my friends. I'm tired of berating myself and hating myself every time my 'mis-management' makes me ill.

I'm tired of fighting that cruel voice within me that tells me I really am making it all up, that they are all right – I am that selfish, that messed up that I would willingly do this to all who love me so much.

I'm tired of pushing through to silence that voice, only to be thrown back into guilt as the effects of pushing my body too hard take hold.

I'm tired of trying to control the uncontrollable.

The effort of doing this alone is killing me, and I'm tired. I can't do it anymore.

You are my hope – one day I will be well. You promise that. After this life there will be no more death or mourning or crying or pain – you will make everything new.

There will be no more sickness. A new body. And until then you are my hope for purpose in this, for comfort amidst the pain, for sustaining and for strength. Strength beyond my own capacity. My strength is spent, I've run out and I need yours.

Thank you for your patience with me Lord. Thank you for your understanding. You know this is hard for me, and you understand why it's hard for me to trust. I don't see your bigger picture and I don't always understand the whys of my circumstances. You get that and you don't condemn me for it.

You have been gentle with me and patient when I was silent, when I refused to talk to you.

You have listened and loved me when I have shouted and raged at you. In my anger, you have loved.

And as my anger has started to subside, you have still been there, loving me and listening to my honest questions, my hurt and confusion. Being patient again as I take small, faltering steps towards you, as I learn to trust again.

Your answer hasn't been healing, you haven't taken my sickness away and you haven't exactly explained why.

Instead you have given me family and friends to support me and help me. They have been your hands and feet, cooking meals, cleaning, caring for my girls and for me.

Instead you have provided for me through a great job for my husband that not only pays for the basics, but also for some help for me, and you gave him an understanding boss who is supportive in our circumstances.

Instead you have given me a new joy in reading your word. You have spoken to me as I've read the Bible. You have brought it to life, helping me to see your heart behind the story and helping me to see your heart for me through it too.

Instead you have given me role models, people who have gone before. Who have walked, and are walking, the path of life-long illness and disability. People who have struggled and strived and raged and tired, and who have learnt to trust you and have experienced your faithfulness, even though their circumstances remain unchanged.

Instead you have given me enough health to live the life you intend for me, to be blessed and to be a blessing.

Instead you are giving me peace, you are restoring my joy in you, and I love you more.

I still don't know why you have given me this particular pain, why me and not others. I also don't know why others suffer more than me in so many different ways. The whys of pain and suffering are not easily answered in this life. I still don't know what the future holds and I'm still afraid, but as I learn to give the control of my life back to you, I am gradually finding that the fear is lessened. The uncertainty of my life is easier to bear in the context of the certainty of the God I know, and am getting to know better as I lean toward him and ask for help.

I have said:

'My way is hidden from the Lord; my cause is disregarded by my God.'

Do you not know? Have you not heard?

The Lord is the everlasting God, the creator of the ends of the earth.

He will not grow tired or weary, and his understanding no-one can fathom.

He gives strength to the weary and increases the power of the weak

Even youths grow tired and weary, and young men stumble and fall, but those who hope in the Lord will renew their strength.

They will soar on wings like eagles, the will run and not grow weary, they will walk and not be faint.

(Isaiah chapter 40 verse 27, The Bible)

My Lord and my God, I want to love you for who you are, not just for what you can do for me.

I know you will never leave me, you have already saved me from the greatest danger I face – that of being lost to you –

you have forgiven me and prepared a place for me in heaven where I will be perfect and healed and whole and with you. Until then Lord, you know the struggle I face, the pain I bear. You know it like no other can. You know what I bear today, and you know what I will have to bear tomorrow. Sustain me, please. Give me the strength I need to keep fighting each day. Comfort me when I weep, hold me when I rage, when I am afraid, please show me that you have not abandoned me and give me courage.

Sick or well, we will all face death in the end; whatever my circumstances please help me to live well, to please you and to end my life in peace so that I can know the joy of being with you face-to-face.

With a full heart and trembling hand I give myself to you, with all my love and all my life.

Your daughter and your friend x

To my nearest and dearest,

      I wish you could understand how lonely it feels to be ill, day in, day out, stuck in the house, isolated, no friends, no phone calls because I can't cope with them, little emails because increasingly I can't cope with them either. I wish you could understand how much I'd like to see you, how you can brighten my day, how you're all I've got now, how you flitting in and out of my life is so hurtful. Small glimpses of you, breezing in and out, watching your back as you walk away back to your busy life. I won't be here forever; I worry you'll regret your lack of caring for me once I've gone.

I wish you would ask me about how my illness affects me, with care and without judgement. I wish you would read my posts and shares on Facebook that explain so much. I wish you wouldn't argue with me about how I manage my illness and tell me I just have to co-operate. Shame on you for being so judgemental and not finding out about ME after all these endless years, but instead bullying me to do what you think I should be doing.

Shame on you all for not taking me / ME seriously.

Sue.

To my family,

> Thank you.

Thank you for being here every step. Thank you for pushing for people to help me, when I had no energy to fight for help myself. Thank you for accepting me, whatever state I'm in, and for picking up the pieces all the times when this illness got too much.

Thank you for helping me move forward, and sharing my achievements with me. And thank you for spending so much time with me, never-ending love and support, regardless of the fact this illness took a lot away from you also.

Thank you x

Dear Friends...

Dear friends,

Life has been more than complicated for me over the past four years. Although I may seem my same old self and look the same, I still am, but I'm battling this horrendous illness called ME. I know you will probably ask what that is, and all I can say is imagine this:

Every day is a complete struggle from day to night.

Constant headaches bashing away at you constantly.

Fatigue that feels like you have the flu and have done twenty marathons at the same time but you will never feel refreshed again, so you feel this day in, day out.

Having no temperature control, so that you have to pile on all the layers possible because you're freezing and then have to take them all off again the next minute because you are boiling.

Having no energy that sometimes the thought of doing something as simple as brushing your teeth is such a daunting prospect.

Having your life changed from one spectrum (being active) to the other (being so inactive) so that you suffer muscle weakness.

Having to use a wheelchair because the legs you were born with can no longer support your weight and the pain is so unbearable.

Being so noise sensitive that a quiet chat sounds like shouting.

Being so sensitive to light that your eyes feel like they are burning.

These are the minority of things that I go through on a daily basis, and I wanted to share this with you as although I still look the same, I have an invisible illness that is exacerbated by the smallest of things. It doesn't mean I should be treated differently but just be treated equally and be understood when having to cancel plans. Things change day-to-day so I can no longer plan ahead but have to take each day as it comes.

Thank you for respecting me and understanding.

Xxxxxxxx

Dear friends,

These last few weeks have been hard and have taken some of you by shock, so imagine how I feel. I really did think I may have cracked this illness. It's as if it thought 'right, let's teach her a lesson, she cannot ignore me'.

Let me explain; I have been feeling so much better. I have had better energy levels and have been able to do more over a longer period of time.

I had been doing some small housework jobs that day and had plans for the evening to go out for a meal. I had a lovely bath and got ready. At the restaurant I ordered my meal and a drink and all was fine. It was a lovely, relaxed atmosphere, with a female vocalist singing and playing the guitar in the corner. Half-way through my soup I started shaking and was having trouble to get spoon to mouth; by the time main course arrived I could not even pick up the salt. To cut a long story short, after a call to speak to an on-call doctor I ended up in a blue-light ambulance and was admitted to the specialist stroke unit.

I was well looked after in some ways, but not in other ways. I had a CT scan which showed nothing, blood tests which showed nothing significant, so after a few days and no improvement I had an MRI scan which was clear. The medics could not understand why I was still showing symptoms but all tests were coming back clear. I had reduced feeling in my right arm and leg. I was moved into a stroke rehab centre and put in a side room, and then started to improve a little as I was getting some sleep. Stroke rehab was not what I needed, but the only way a person with ME can get to the help and services i.e. physiotherapy and occupational therapy that I needed as an in-patient. After twelve days in hospital I am now home, still having difficulties but improving. I think this has been a sharp learning curve for us all; you need to respect the illness and learn to work with the illness and not against it.

I want to say thank you to my friends who have stood by me. One thing I would like to know is why it has taken a bad turn like this for some of you to understand that I am ill. I am sure some of you thought I was just saying I had ME for attention and sympathy which I don't need or want. Thank you to those of you who have been at my side from the beginning throughout - it has been a long eight years.

xx

To my friends who have stayed,

You would have been perplexed by this, my sudden departure. Peculiar symptoms that you couldn't understand. My change in personality to one of a sudden despairing invalid. Some of you have only known me as one having illness, never seeing me well; but when severe ME hit it was like a new condition in itself.

Confused you may be, but you choose to take my word for it, stay with me even when I can't have you near, or when I can't reply or respond in any way. You've stood by me and stand there still, and didn't leave like some. With you, it's not out of sight, out of mind, but you enquire after me, knowing the response yet asking anyway and taking the reply.

You give, not passing pity, but real empathy and compassion. Trying to grasp what it's like for me, genuinely wanting to know, to share my fraught life. Wishing you could take it from me, even offering to swap your health at times.

Little presents through the post, cards, and short messages. Words of encouragement which may sound clumsy to you but to me so completely honest and meaningful. Often you need not even say or do anything; I know that you are there.

I hold absolute appreciation and gratitude for you all, and I hope one day I can be the one standing by your side.

M x

Dear friends,

I know that ME is something that you might not be able to understand that well, so I'm writing this letter to help you see what it is like and for you to know how to help me best.

First of all, even though I have ME, I'm not unable to do EVERYTHING, just sometimes I can't do one thing because I've chosen to do another and have to prioritise. Please don't feel like you can't invite me to places with you. You aren't making me feel awkward by asking me and me not being able to come. I will honestly do my best to do things with you and I try really hard to not say 'no', although I know it must feel like that's my answer every time. It's nothing personal; it's just me trying to manage my ME because sometimes just getting through every day is hard enough.

Sometimes you are really over-protective of me and I really do thank you for how much you care, but sometimes I need you to take a step back. I am still human and sometimes I do just get a bug like healthy people, and although it does mess up my ME symptoms and make them worse, sometimes you tell me what to do as though I'm having a full-blown relapse. Please don't take this as a criticism of you because you're great, but I know my own body; I know the signs and signals and sometimes it isn't the ME causing the main issue. If I'm off work, it could just be that I have a bug - it doesn't mean that I can't cope with my job or that I need to consider sick leave by any means. I know you do it out of concern but sometimes it feels like you are pressuring me to admit defeat when actually it's not that serious after all.

If I have to use things to help me get around, like my wheelchair, please don't treat me any differently. Please make the same jokes we always do and have the same little laughs like usual. Don't feel the need to be over-nice to me; I haven't done anything amazing or anything that deserves that sort of treatment. And if other people see you treating me like a normal person then they won't feel so awkward or embarrassed around me, and I won't feel awkward or embarrassed around them. Which will mean that I'll feel more confident going out with you and doing things! I haven't had to use my wheelchair for the last couple of years and I'm trying very hard to keep it that way - but if I ever do need it, it doesn't mean my personality has changed or that you need to feel sorry for me.

When I am having a bad day, please don't be offended if I don't feel like seeing you or talking to you. It's not that I don't enjoy your company or that you've done anything wrong. When I'm having a bad day I shut myself away and drown out as much going on around me as possible because any little thing takes up so much of my energy, even talking, and I want to save it all so much because I want to get back on my feet as quickly as I can. I will always make sure we have a chance to catch up when I'm feeling a bit better!

You are brilliant and I don't want you to feel like this is a dig at you. I hope this helps you to understand a little bit what it's like for me.

Thank you.

Jasmine xxxxxxxx

To the three wise men,

Many times when you have a serious illness like ME, where you can't even lift your head off the pillows, your friends who you work with just go by the way side. Yeah it's a bit difficult to take - but they don't owe you anything. However the friends, some who have been there since before you could walk, don't want to know you - and years later they say 'I just didn't know it was that bad, I had no idea'. No excuses I'm afraid, although no grudges borne - life is too short for that.

However, all the above is unhelpful - the amazing thing about this illness is the ones that did stick around. You never knew about the illness, but you were there for my four years of being bed-bound, the next sixteen years of varying degrees of health. I know I can trust you with my life.

When I could hardly remember your names or hold a conversation, all my confidence and dignity sapped waiting for death, hoping to die to get out of this 'life'. But you guys kept saying 'you will get better, you will get better', and we all know no-one believed that.

You have all known me as a child, then into a fit and robust young man who worked hard and played sports whenever time was free. It all must have come as a shock when I just fell. Many didn't believe me, but all of you know me so well that it didn't even enter your head that I wasn't unwell.

Over the years I began to get better and met another ME sufferer who was to change my life; I know you three wise men supported me.

A decision had to be made when me and Miranda decided to get married who was going to be my best man. For some reason, and not because I put one of you above another, I don't, but it was an easy decision to make. I picked you

Spencer, closer than many brothers; it always has felt we weren't just friends but blood.

The path unfortunately since marriage has been a harsh one. Everything was good until I lost my mother and Miranda became bed-bound. I was in a complete state, many times contemplating suicide as the only way out of this torture. It seemed the logical solution, but again my three wise men came to my rescue.

I owe so much to you Dennis, to you Gary and to you Spencer - including my life.

Nigel

Kieran,

I am glad to hear you are recovering from flu and are feeling a bit better.

You have always said you wished you could understand what it really felt like for me, living with ME. I reckon you might be in a good place today, as you start to recover, to at least understand better the fatigue and pain I experience on a daily basis. It will be harder to describe what it's like living with a condition that refuses to follow a set trajectory, not allowing me to plan like you and the rest of my friends. It took me by surprise too; it coaxed and teased and then hit with such ferocity that I was bullied into submission and had no option but to succumb.

I just laughed off your 'lazy' jokes but this has not been easy - this condition has changed my life. I know you were relieved when I could talk to you or text you; you would tease that I was 'in the land of the living' and occasionally you would post me those all-important chocolate bars. But I don't think you really understood.

You were less tolerant when I didn't respond to your tweets or call you for weeks at a time and there were times I thought our friendship wouldn't survive the test, just like some others.

To begin with I couldn't even sit unaided; every movement was unbearable. Remember how I moaned when I had to sip those horrible energy drinks - but when I look at the few photos my sisters took at this time I don't even recognise myself, I was just skin and bones. I looked and felt like the living dead. And there are still too many days when I have those blinding headaches that rob me of my other senses, days when I am overcome with breathlessness or chest pains and just sitting up can cause me to faint repeatedly. Poor Mum and Dad were frantic. I cannot ever remember writing a letter before, unless it was for a school project; but I think in writing this I can better understand their concerns! My new Irish Dancing dress hung on that wardrobe door for months; I insisted, I desperately wanted to think myself better.

I have tried to explain that completing everyday tasks are still like a military operation to me. I mean, I'm often exhausted before breakfast, even on a good day. I have to micro-manage everything, like getting ready for school which can be daunting. It starts when I wake up and continues with the pain of getting out of bed, choosing clothes, showering, brushing my hair, putting clothes on and adjusting to their weight on my aching body, choosing breakfast and eating breakfast. Some days I feel that I should attempt to find ways to make my hair look better and hide the patches on my skull where alopecia has attacked. I try to cover the black shaded areas under my tired eyes but some days I have to give up and crawl back to bed. I struggle to pack a bag and get out the front door to the car. Sometimes just the noise and chatter of my sisters on the school run or the radio being too loud can drain me of all my energy, and the day is lost.

I worry, even now that I am getting better and spending more time out of bed, getting back to school and normal life, that I catch a cold or become unwell. I worry about that uncontrollable, unrelenting downward spiral robbing me of everything again. When you have ME, being prepared for the worst is part of the day. I miss the freedom associated with youth.

I don't know if I ever thanked you out loud Kieran but you helped save me with your idle chatter and silly jokes, you kept me in touch with what was going on in the outside world. I'm so glad that you are feeling better, flu is horrible but at least you know the effects will be short-lived. I hope you enjoy the chocolate bar!

Collette

To my friends,

Before I got ill, I was just like you. I was young and energetic - I loved nothing more than meeting up with you and enjoying some of the best (and funniest) moments of my life so far. Can you remember when we all finished school and went on holiday before starting uni? We were out doing things every day and in the pub every night, and when the pub closed we sat round in our pyjamas chatting and laughing all night. And even when we all went away, we'd meet up in the holidays and do it all again. It meant everything to me.

When I got ill it completely shattered my world.

I didn't know what was going on with me, but despite what the doctors were telling me I knew that something wasn't right. Being so young you'd expect to bounce back from a virus very quickly, but for some reason I just didn't. I just got more and more ill, and as you know I was eventually diagnosed with ME. It became a battle just to get to my lectures. I stopped going out in the evenings. I managed to get through; I got myself to my lectures and managed to join a couple of societies, but I never went on any of the socials. I'd spend hours at home thinking of everyone out having fun and wishing I was there too. Life for me was never the same again.

Did you ever give up on me? Not once! You were always so understanding and made so much effort to keep in touch. After finishing my course I became severely ill and had to put my further plans on hold. By that time, you all had your first jobs and were settling in, making new friends. Did you ever forget about me? Never. You still kept in touch and came to visit me either in hospital or at home loads. And when you were with me, you didn't focus on my illness, you focused on me. You focused on updating me with all the gossip and with making me laugh. You could not have made me feel more loved if you'd tried. When I was too ill to come to birthday parties, you brought them to me all in a way that I could manage. I still have the card from one party I'd missed that you made me, with a picture of you all with 'we love you' written underneath.

I want to thank you from the bottom of my heart for taking the time to do all that for me. Thank you for still inviting me to things even though you know I won't be able to make it. It makes me feel valued - it makes me feel like I am so much more than an ME sufferer. I'm a lot better than I was, and six years after becoming ill, I'm slowly learning to manage my condition. Sometimes I can come out with you but thank you for understanding when I leave early. Thank you for not handling me with kid-gloves, but for letting me get stuck in and have a laugh, even if I can't manage it for very long. Thank you for understanding that I need time to rebuild my strength when we've done something.

And last of all, and most importantly, thank you so much for always believing me - for believing that my symptoms are real and that I have a physical, not psychological condition. People are so quick to judge, to not understand and to think that because they can't see it, it's either not there or it's in my head. Society passes ME off as a 'fake' condition - an excuse not to work or to just whinge and take the easy route through life. But you have never ever done any of that. Actually, you've always highlighted my achievements and recognised that I am trying my absolute best in life. That means more than I could ever put into words.

They say that many people walk through our lives, but true friends leave footprints on our hearts. I'll never forget just how amazing you have all been, and continue to be.

So much love,
Your very grateful friend.

XxxxX

To my former classmate/ friend,

You tell me that I'm lucky, but I'm not. I spend all day exhausted, in pain, and feeling so sick I might cry. I may not go to school, but that doesn't make me lucky. I don't go to school because I physically can't. I don't have the energy, or the strength. Does that me lucky? Not being able to get an education?

You also say you want ME so that you won't have to go to school. But trust me, you don't want this illness. You'll cry at least once a day, have to go to a hospital at least twice a week and have to deal with all the symptoms. You'll see your friends about once every two months, and when you do see them, you'll only get to talk to them for about a minute, or maybe two (if you're feeling good). Any longer than that, and you'll have payback for the next few days.

When I'm not at school, you tell people my illness is when I 'just get tired'. ME is a lot more than just being tired. I have a headache that never goes away, not even with medication and complete silence. I feel so sick that the thought of eating anything repulses me. My legs hurt too much to walk, I have to go out in a wheelchair, and my arms feel so heavy and ache so much that even picking up a really light cup half-full of water drains all the energy from me. Sometimes, I get a large lump in my throat that makes it hard to breathe. So tell me, does all this sound like just being tired?

You're always complaining about the strict teachers, the teachers who can't actually teach, the annoying boys who never shut up and the popular girls who have faces caked in make-up. I used to complain about them too, but now I actually miss them. I miss the lessons where everyone got told off for the smallest things, and the ones where no-one got told off, even if we were all extremely loud and disruptive. I miss the boys who made cheesy jokes and called everyone 'gay'. I miss the girls who bitched about people behind their backs, and had friendships as complicated as the plot of *A Midsummer Night's Dream*.

You're the lucky one, you know. You're getting the chance to make friends, get an education, and, if you work hard enough, the qualifications needed to get a decent job. I didn't know I was lucky before I got ME, but now I realise how lucky I was. You have a life, a good one. So next time you call someone lucky, please make sure you know all the real facts, not just one; they don't go to school. Also, please don't take your life for granted. Appreciate your friends, teachers, school and health. Not everyone has those things. And if you do have those things, it can all be taken away from you with one simple diagnosis.

From Esther

To my school friends,

      I wish I had talked to you about my ME more. I didn't want to be boring or sound like I was attention seeking so I never said anything unless you asked. It was only when I was older that I realised you probably never asked because you didn't know if I wanted to talk about it.

I should have told you that my ME left me feeling exhausted, that for a few weeks I was practically bed-bound and for months I was housebound and didn't even go outside into the garden. Most days I didn't even have the energy to get dressed and just lay on the sofa in my pyjamas. I suffered from nausea, shaking, dizziness, headaches, sleep disturbance, brain fog, difficulty concentrating and sensitivity to light and sounds. Imagine having flu all the time. It's not just tiredness. It's like being a malfunctioning battery; it takes a long time for my energy to charge up and then it runs down quickly. I might have looked OK when you saw me, but once my energy ran out I looked and felt awful. I was probably far more ill than you ever realised.

I tried hard to stay in touch with you all, but only a few of you were supportive. To start with it was like I was the centre of attention and then the novelty of me being ill for so long wore off. It felt like I was always the one putting the effort in. I was only well enough to send a couple of texts on good days so I had practically no social life. It meant so much to me when one friend got everyone to sign a get well card for me. I still have it.

When I recovered enough to be able to meet up with you sometimes things were easier. I really enjoyed having a few of you over to my house and it was a real treat to be well enough to go to the cinema as it was the only outing I could manage to do. Then one friend complained that all we ever did was go to the cinema and couldn't we do something else. I can't explain the hollow, empty feeling I got when she said this to me. I just enjoyed being able to spend time with you all.

I felt so upset and betrayed when I found out some of you had organised get-togethers and not invited me. One friend told me people had said 'she won't be well enough to go anyway so what's the point of inviting her?' It was awful not being able to go out and do things, but I would have so much preferred that it was because I wasn't well enough to go, rather than because people didn't bother to invite me. It made it so much worse. I stopped inviting one girl to things I organised after she'd had a party and invited all our friends and nearly the whole of the rest of the year, but not me. She never got in touch with me so I assumed she didn't want to be friends. She was then very upset that I stopped inviting her to things and got a friend to ask me why. I couldn't believe it.

Sometimes I felt like a circus attraction. When I started trying to go back into school a bit, people who I hardly knew would flock round asking me questions. I knew that later they'd be talking about me with their friends. I hated to think about what people were saying about me behind my back. I was shy and hated being the focus of so much attention. I just wanted to be left alone and to have a few hours of being 'normal' with my friends.

Some of you were wonderful. Even small gestures meant the world to me. One friend said that if I told her what I wanted to do and who I wanted to invite then she'd organise a meet up for me. I was so grateful. Just the fact that she offered made me feel so happy. We're still friends today.

I wish I'd had the courage to drop many of you as friends. I know that sounds awful, but I used up so much energy trying to stay in touch with all of you when I should have picked my best friends and spent my energy on them. I was too afraid of offending you, which is ridiculous when the problem was that you had too little regard for my feelings. I was surprised which of you were understanding. Having ME made me realise who my real friends are.

Sarah xxxxx

To my amazing friend (hopefully you'll know who you are by the time you finish reading this!),

        I first met you two years ago now. I got to know you because you saw past the ME and gave me a chance - a chance that others may not have wanted to give me - and for that I can't thank you enough, because it opened doors for me.

In the last couple of years I've come to realise that I don't think I've ever come across anyone so understanding and supportive about my ME as you.

At first, I didn't want to tell you about my illness because I was scared about what you, and others, would think. I wanted to get to know you first, (if I was going to tell you about it at all) and for you to get to know me as a person too. And I liked the feeling of being normal; I liked the thought that to you, I was exactly the same as everybody else.

I couldn't keep it up. I got a virus which aggravated my symptoms, so had to tell you eventually. I don't know what I was worrying about! You were so lovely, you believed me and you never treated me any differently for it. It was like you'd known all along, and that helped me a lot. I wasn't met with the awkward responses I usually get; 'ME... isn't that where you get tired all the time?' or 'I know someone who had that. They changed their diet, started exercising and did meditation and now they're cured!'

You have always been there, pretty much instantly from that moment on - whilst I spent the following weekend lying in bed feeling really ill, you kept in touch and rang and texted me loads to see if I was OK. I knew then that I was safe, I was really lucky to have you, and I had (and still have) so much respect for you for how much you helped me.

Over the last couple of years, you've seen me through plenty of ups and downs and you have always been a rock, solidly there for me, knowing exactly what to say and what to do during the bad times. I really appreciate how you are always honest and open with me, and allow me to see things that I might not have considered before. I know that you mean everything you say and that I can always trust you; I know you always have my best interests at heart. But you are also someone who is a complete ray of sunshine and can cheer me up in seconds! You have had me in absolute stitches and it's little moments like those that I hold on to so much when I'm having a bad time. After all, they do say that laughter is the best form of medicine!

You also give me so much confidence and strength to fight for things myself. You encourage me and help me to believe in myself, to recognise what I can do, and I can never put into words just how much that kind of support helps me to live my day-to-day life when I have to face things that aren't always easy. However, you've always known when I need a little bit of help to fight my corner. For that I am so grateful, and I hope you know that if the tables were turned I'd do the same for you.

I've had to make some very tough decisions over the past year and times have been a bit uncertain to say the least, but it has been massively helpful that you have talked to me so much about it all and have constantly reassured me that I've made the right decision - and that things will be OK. I feel a lot better than I would have done without all of that. I completely believe you when you tell me that everything will be OK and you inspire me to make things not just OK, but absolutely amazing and let a lot of good come from all this suffering. You've helped me to accept my condition and the limitations that come with it, and have helped me to look at ways of working around my ME whilst living my dream at the same time. Thank you for helping me to come to terms with it all and for making me see that there is nothing wrong with re-thinking my plans because of my situation. I'm now in a place where, thanks to you, I'm seeing this as something really exciting... something that I'd never have discovered if it hadn't been for the ME forcing me to step back, and something that I believe I'll enjoy so much more than my original plans. I'm just so honoured that I'll get to share all of the exciting things that are going to happen with you.

I know I'm a pain, but you never allow me to feel like I am one. Even though we joke about you nagging me, I love it when you do because it really helps me! You just seem to understand, even without having ME yourself; I don't need to tell you how much I hate having ME especially at my age, but you never make me feel anything less than completely valued... and normal. And that makes everything feel better. I don't worry about whether people believe me or understand my illness, because I know that you do and that you are always there... and that's all that matters.

Thank you for all of your love and care, for always knowing what to do, for letting me moan about the same thing time and time again and for always listening (just getting it off my chest helps me so much). Thank you for making time for me even though your life is so busy, for knowing exactly what I mean when I talk about a 'thingy bob' or a 'whatsit' (brain fog is amazing), for not minding about where we eat as I can't eat gluten (and for giving me the most amazing gluten-free cookbook in the world!). Thank you for being there, giving advice and looking after me when I'm ill, for getting me things and coming to the hospital for me, and for offering a safe and calm space at yours when things get too much. Thank you for just being who you are. You're one in a trillion and mean a lot to me. Don't ever underestimate how much you've helped me get through.

We've had a lot of fun times as well as the not-so-fun ones, and I know there are plenty more good times to come. I'm really looking forward to them all. I love you to bits and I hope you know that I am always here for you too - and always ready to do whatever I can to help you out!

And you're right - there is more to me than this illness... so thank you for showing me that!

I am sending you a massive hug and hoping you've worked out who I am... and that this letter is aimed at you!

Loads and loads of love and hugs xxxx

Dear friends,

Without you I would not be where I am; it's a cliché but it's true. You're the people who help me smile, help me laugh, help me cry, help me calm down, help me relax, help me stay strong, help me through. You're the people who I could call at any time of the day and I know you would be there for me. But you're no ordinary friends. You're all going through the same thing as I am.

When I first got ill I was so lost and helpless. I was frightened of all the dark that was surrounding me and having no friends to battle it with. But then along you came, and from that moment I knew I would never be alone. We didn't make friends in the normal way, we did it backwards really. They say never meet someone who you've only talked to over the internet; now, if I had followed that advice, I would truly be alone, because nearly all of my friends now I have met off the internet.

Sometimes I do still feel alone because you are all so far away, and with the nature of this illness we can't see each other that much. But all I have to do is text and you're there for me. You actually don't realise how much you mean to me and how much you have helped me through. We have a bond that no-one else can have unless you're going through the same thing, the same illness. And because we have this bond it means that no matter where we are we will always have each other.

So I just wanted to thank you, because I have lost a lot of friends with this illness but then if I hadn't have lost them I wouldn't have gained all of you! I want to THANK YOU for being my friend, for putting up with everything I do, texting me every day and supporting me to achieve my goals. With you as my friends, I know I can conquer anything. You all inspire me every day with how you cope with everything life throws at you. You're my inspirations, my heroes.

You know who you are.

Love,

Sophie xxxx

Dear Sufferers...

A note to those who have recovered,

>Please remember those of us who are left behind, the ones who are still struggling everyday with pain, exhaustion and frustration. Those whose recovery is taking years despite how careful we are, how well we pace ourselves or the treatments we try. We don't want recovery any less than you, we just aren't as lucky.

We are pleased that you are doing better, and it gives us hope that one day, we will get better too; but hope will only get you so far, then we have to settle down to the endurance of our day-to-day existence.

There are people with ME who have been ill for over a decade and in that time have seen so many people come and go. Watched as their friends have recovered and moved on, leaving them behind along with the memories of their illness.

The feeling of abandonment hurts, especially when you've put time and energy into supporting that person whilst they were ill. We don't expect you to contact us every day, or even every week; but the occasional card or text would be nice, and try to remember what we are still going through. Tell us how you are doing; but don't forget to ask how we are, what we are up to and how life is in general.

It may be hard to be reminded of what you've been through; but the person still suffering needs the support, now more than ever, and as they were there for you, please be there for them.

This isn't meant to be a guilt trip or to point the finger of blame, just a plea to remember the ones still on the long, slow road to recovery.

C xx

To mild or moderate ME sufferers,

Firstly, let me say that by using the terms 'mild' or 'moderate', I am in no way trying to downplay how much you suffer. What is termed 'mild' or 'moderate' in the ME world would be classed as 'severe' in some other illnesses. I know things are hard, and that quality of life can be massively affected by mild or moderate ME– but I also know from bitter experience that things can be much, much harder.

My purpose in writing this letter is to say please be careful and guard your health. If I were in your position, I wouldn't want to know about those who are more severe than me, wouldn't want to think about how severe this illness can get. And I wouldn't want to be careful all the time; I'd want to push the boat out at least occasionally whilst I could. However...

Everything is a question of weighing up risks versus benefits of an activity. You absolutely have the right to push the boat out, make your own choices, etc. But the problem is, ME doesn't care about your human rights. And it can't do maths; sometimes 2 + 2 + ME will equal four; sometimes it'll equal forty-five, or whatever. The only consistent thing about ME is that it's a [four letter word], and that it'll only get worse if you're not careful. If you overdo things, maybe you'll get lucky and be back to your normal level after a few weeks' rest - and I really hope that's the case. But on the other hand, you might not be lucky, and it may take you months, years or longer to recover. I really hope that doesn't happen to you. But so many of us can look back and see things that seemed so important/ unavoidable at the time, which we now hugely regret doing because we're still suffering the worsening of our condition years later. I'm nowhere near as severe as many others - but still I have to weigh up the risks of apparently small activities, such as having a wash or brushing my hair on days when I am physically capable of doing those things. I did not realise the damage I was doing to my body when I was mild/moderate, as I had not yet been diagnosed so did not understand the disease. I was denied the chance to be careful. Please listen to your body while you have the chance. (I'm sorry to sound so harsh and preachy, but this is a harsh disease, and I would be failing you as a fellow human being if I didn't tell you the truth. There are no easy/nice answers to ME; if there were, we'd all be healthy and out living life to the full.)

I wish you all the best, and truly hope you never have to suffer the devastation of severe ME.

Xxx

This is an open letter to anyone affected directly or indirectly by ME:

This isn't a scientific text, nor is it a guide to anything. It is merely my story, about me and ME. Whilst I do enjoy writing it is usually fiction, particularly short stories, which absorb my time and always have. This is probably due to my attention span and a bit of laziness, combined with a fear of 'waffling on' too much. Be that as it may, I have never tried writing non-fiction so I'm going to make this up as I go along, which handily, is also my process for writing fiction!

These notes are a sort of diary, although not very date specific, about who I was, who I am now, what's changed and how it changed me. Please don't expect any miracle cures or medicinal insight. I'm not entirely sure of even my purpose for writing this, other than to tell you, dear reader, that you are not alone.

Maybe you have ME, maybe you don't, maybe someone close to you does, or not. Maybe you were emptying a bin and found this - I don't know, but I promise you my sole intention is to explain myself, my life and to hopefully be of some use to someone out there.

At first...

This part of the story starts a little before things get bad. Imagine, if you will, a Scooby Doo memory sequence where the screen goes wavy:

It's 2012, it's August and I have just finished a summer of temping work. It's been one of the best jobs I can remember having (there have been quite a few), scanning geological data with a great bunch of people. I'm sad it has to end but I have another temp job to go to.

'Temp job?' I hear you say. Yes. Basically I finished my HND in Manufacturing Engineering in July 2011 and couldn't get a related job that didn't involve getting spat on all day. That's probably something to do with politics that I can't be bothered to try and understand.

The second temp job was in a book warehouse picking orders. It was about six miles from home with a massive great hill in between. I should point out here that in May 2012 I turned thirty-two and I had a few hobbies:

Weightlifting - three times per week.

Cycling - fifty miles per week.

Football - five-a-side once per week.

Dog walking - two to three miles, three to four times per week.

Running - sometimes with the dogs, once per week.

Beer, TV and Xbox are also featured, but not enough to be too relevant.

So, running round a warehouse slinging books about was no challenge to me. I felt indestructible. I wasn't a body-beautiful sculpted person, I'm 5'4 and stocky, but I could bench press my own body weight. I was proportionately big but fit as well.

Then...

The temp job lived up to its name and dried up as expected, though I can't remember when. I do remember that in October I interviewed at a place that makes parts for planes for a position on the shop floor. All my previous engineering interviews had stated a lack of 'hands on experience', so I thought the plane job would get that part resolved. I interviewed well and started the following Monday as a temp-to-perm employee (basically, don't be an idiot and we'll take you on).

[Hurrah! Stick this out for eighteen months and then start job hunting again. You'll be on easy street in no time, son!]

That was what I told myself so I knuckled down to learn. I went into model employee mode; always early, fastidiously polite, asking for more when I was done, etc. There was only one problem; I sucked at the job. It was a delicate process dealing with wax and some REALLY heavy tools. Now, everyone laughed when I told my friends what I was doing, working with a material so fragile. They all know what I am to gentle - uninitiated, comical. There was another thing, I kept coming home tired. I'd walk to work, walk back, do a sporting hobby and go to bed. At weekends I'd sleep for twelve hours easily. The tiredness was nearly always compounded so by Friday I'd want to cry. It made me EVEN worse at my job!

It got to a point where I was costing the company too much money to keep trashing the stuff I made so I was moved onto a 'robust' area. This was around January 2013. Equally as heavy but there was nearly no delicacy needed. Relief! Sweet relief! I could do this job, and I could do it well. The boss man would walk up every now and then to see how I was doing and it was all smiles. At first.

Then, after a couple of weeks, I found that I was feeling shattered at work. My boss would see me slumped on the table while I was waiting for the press to fill the die. After he commented a couple of times I decided to speak to my GP. I don't really remember the course of events but I had loads of blood tests which came back negative, whilst my symptoms got worse. I gave up running, still no joy. I gave up cycling, wrecked. Stopped weights, flat as a pancake. Finally gave up my beloved footy and still no better. All it changed was that I was coming home and sleeping from 6pm through to 6am with no sport to get in the way.

Eventually the boss moved me onto another department where the workload was very light, but it was dull. Dull as hell. Awful. But it was still a wage, and hopefully the doctor could fix me - then I'd get back to my eighteen month plan. This process of various tests, specialists and fatigue carried on until May, when I was very lucky. My wife took me to Barcelona for my birthday present and we had an exceptional three-day break. I came back into work on the Friday to find out I'd been laid off. The company had outsourced the boring job I was doing to some poor sod in parts unknown. This was a bit of a blow, but I took positive action and called the agency that had been so good to me. As luck would have it, they had a position free in an out-of-hours call centre where I had worked before and I could start next week. I knew the shifts would be random and unsociable but the money was good for very little effort, plus I knew and liked the other workers. What this ended up meaning was that I was sleeping all day, working in the evening and then going back to bed, and these were only four hour shifts.

I was still seeing the doctor as my symptoms had amiably made room amongst their number for joint and muscle pain. Pain with no previous effort or impact to cause it. I had also had mild and infrequent confusion but ignored it as 'being dizzy'. The doctor (who has been magnificent) prescribed various ibuprofen type tablets and gels, but I'd found that I was up at maximum dose with no relief, and my stomach started to give me searing pain (a juicy side effect of OD'ing the Neurofen). I was given co-codamol and it was just keeping my pain at bay.

It was also during this time that I started to experience total 'power outages' as I called them. If you're old enough to remember vinyl, it's like listening to a record but turning the power off while it's still spinning. The sound just winds down to a stop. That's similar to how I experience these outages; my wife calls them 'wobbles', as in 'you look a little grey, are you having a wobble?' If you don't remember vinyl, please ask someone with ME who is better at explaining things than me! Alongside the energy falling away, I feel hot and/ or cold, sweaty, very weak, and sometimes terrified.

It was about the second or third one I'd had that was a few hours before a shift, and my wife put me to bed and called in saying I wasn't going to make it. The next day my GP signed me off sick and we began to seriously raise the subject of ME. She said that I would have to jump through some NHS hoops to rule out any other possible ailments and she would work out an agenda so that we could go from there. A couple of weeks later I received a letter asking to arrange my first appointment with the rheumatologist. During this time I had also started the process of claiming ESA as I was signed off, although not from any given employer as I'd been working through an agency, which doesn't have any sort of sick pay.

This marked a whole new chapter in my life - I'd been unemployed before but never through ill health. My symptoms were developing further, where brain fog was at times (and still is) a real problem. I'd lose words, I'd get confused, I couldn't understand people or if I could I didn't follow it well. I'd make mistakes. A lot of mistakes. I clearly remember an occasion at the supermarket where I wanted a cheap bar of milk chocolate and my wife wanted some dark chocolate for cooking. I tried to pick up three of each but then got caught in a difficult conversation about how many of which type we had left in the cupboard at home. In the end I got annoyed and confused so I grabbed three of each. It wasn't until I got home that I found I'd picked up five milk and one dark. I was so confused when I opened the bag, I thought it was some sort of joke but my wife reassured me that I'd told her I knew what I was doing and picked them correctly, so she left me to it. I was scared by that, it felt like a lurch into senility. I'm grateful to have such lovely, trustworthy people around me.

By the time the rheumatologist appointment came round I had already been going to a hydrotherapy pool. The problem with that was that it flattened me. I mean totally. The day after I would be bed-bound, had to be helped to the bathroom, helped to and in the shower, dressed, food brought to me. All I could do was listen to podcasts and, for a very short time, read. The second day was better as I could get downstairs, but it was the day before the next session by the time I could walk properly again. The rheumatologist proved me to be inflexible but not a patient that could be helped by her department. I had similar pain to what she dealt with but no swollen joints, and my bloods indicated no rheumatic issues. So that was ruled out.

I'd also been having an on-and-off fling with the Clinical Investigations Department concerning sleep apnoea. For anyone who may not know, sleep apnoea is when a sleeping person stops breathing for a period of time during sleep. It reduces the amount of oxygen getting into the blood-stream meaning that the patient feels tired upon waking. It's as if you sleep for eight hours but only feel the benefit of sleeping for half that or less. One way that apnoea is recognised is through sleep study. Oh, how I loved sleep study! Basically, one straps a bunch of equipment to one's torso, a pulse reader on the finger and one of those clear tubes over the ears but under the nose, so that you look like the kid who turned up a fancy dress party as a pretty rubbish Robocop because his parents were drunk again. Now, this setup isn't heavy but it's not comfortable either, and usually I wouldn't wear anything tight-fitting to sleep in. Basically, over a ten-hour study I slept for about two hours and spent the next day in a foul mood, slightly less charming than a grizzly bear on PCP.

There were a few re-runs of this test, and ultimately I was told that I do have apnoea but not sufficiently bad to cause the problems I'm having, and certainly not bad enough to consider surgery or a pump that forces air into your face overnight.

During all of these visits to various hospitals they always took my height, weight and blood pressure. Now, I have a history of high blood pressure problems dating back around ten years, and at one point was in hospital with it and subsequently put on medication. That was a long time ago; I have changed a lot since then including stopping smoking five years ago, moderating my drinking and getting fit. I'd not had any blood pressure issues for more than five years, but since my readings were high before one particular appointment it was flagged as something to look into. What was ignored is that prior to the appointment there was nowhere to park, I'd been stuck behind a complete twit all the way up there and I dislike being prodded and poked by specialists, especially when I was already convinced I had ME, so saw this as futile - hence my elevated readings. The net result of all of this was an overnight blood pressure monitor. For one twenty-four hour period I had to have a box strapped to my chest linked to a blood pressure cuff. Every twenty-five minutes or so the box would kick into life and pump air into the cuff (far tighter than the nurses did, to the point where I'd get pins and needles), hold it for about twenty seconds and then record the readings. This meant no sleep - see aforementioned, drug addled bear.

Next...

It's worth pointing out that during this time I was only receiving ESA which is about £143 per fortnight. I happen to be wonderfully lucky that I have a fantastic and supportive wife who, not only helps me by doing things for me such as driving to collect a prescription or dressing me, but also ensures I keep as upbeat as possible. Taking me out for random drives or just into the supermarket for some milk, helping me get out of the house. She has, throughout this situation, helped me arrange to have my friends over as I can't really go out very much. Whilst doing this, she has also held down a 37.5 hour per week job to keep up our rent, pay the bills, etc. This has also meant that we have had to forgo a lot of luxury items but she has happily adapted without so much as a sniff, so I am eternally grateful to her.

For around ten years I have been dependent on anti-depressants and whilst I regularly have them I am okay. When I stopped work the impact of the situation hit me very hard. Not only could I not earn, I couldn't do any of the stuff I used to love to do like football or cycling. That made me really sad. I'd get frustrated that I used to be able to lift weights with ease, yet now couldn't hang a shirt on a washing line. The sense of loss rang through me and I knew I was on the back foot - this was coupled by an increase in pain. The same random joint and muscle pains, but more intense and lasting for longer. There was now also pain after 'exertion', as in if I walked to the end of the road and back, I would suffer leg, hip and back pain. This was a body that used to cycle three miles to football, play five-a-side for an hour and then cycle back!

So I was, without question, way more depressed than before. My GP gave me an increased dose of my usual citalopram, upped from 20mg to 40mg and she also prescribed tramadol. Tramadol is an opiate; it is in the same family as heroin and as a pain killer it is very effective. It's also addictive so care must be taken. Now, when I wake up in the morning I take one or two tramadol, two co-codamol and two citalopram. Once these are in I have to sit and wait before I can move.

After a short period of time my mood began to level out as a result of the increased dose of citalopram. This was great as I felt I could at least try and face things, and with the tramadol I could even be a little more active. I could get out into the woods with my dogs, which was a real bonus - I'd missed it so much! I couldn't do much, but what I could do I relished. I started doing the dishes and the laundry; it meant I had a purpose, a task every day just like having a job again! Don't get me wrong, I'm ambitious and I want to be doing more than that, but it meant so much to feel useful once more.

Not too long after my new found CV enhancing skill-set increase, I was brought back down to earth with a bump. And then a really good shoeing. I didn't realise that tramadol, when taken in conjunction with co-codamol, results in constipation of epic proportions. I've no real shame left so I'll be frank; I was a twice-a-day man for as long as I could remember, three if I was lucky so I was used to a fairly fast transit time. I didn't notice that I'd stopped opening my bowels until the fourth day when the pain started. I've no idea, dear reader, whether you've had constipation and how bad it may have been, but this was a different level of bad compared to my previous experiences. One Sunday I was happily playing some Xbox (probably on the easiest setting) when I noticed some sharp abdominal pain. Then it suddenly got crazy bad. Bad like a razor wire tapeworm. There was nothing I could do but lay down and cry. I knew straight away that it was constipation and quickly realised it was going to be quite a backlog. My wife rushed out and got me some prune juice and off-the-shelf laxatives, so I set about those in between cramps. I spent the next three hours on and off the loo, wrestling out the tiniest crumbs of rubbish; all the while I was sweating and shuddering with the movement inside. I expect that if I were to ever get shot in the stomach and someone were to then use an electric whisk in the bullet hole, the pain would be comparable. Eventually everything relaxed and I spent the rest of the day eating fruit. Cue the immediate addition of Laxido to my prescription list.

Laxido sounds like a rubbish Spanish game show, one you probably don't want to win. It comes in sachets of powder that are to be mixed with water and drunk. The powder is apparently orange flavour, but it is nasty. It's one that you take it in one go whilst holding your nose. Having said all of that, it is effective and that's the important part.

Up until recently...

Armed with a fully functioning digestive system I can start to bring you through to current times. In January 2014 I had an appointment with a CFS specialist through my GP. Incidentally, I've seen a huge amount on Twitter about the differences between CFS and ME (CFS being Chronic Fatigue Syndrome) and some of it gets quite heated. In this context I'm unsure which way the specialist views it, so I'm calling it all ME/ CFS.

The specialist told me that he thought I had ME/ CFS, and that he wanted to get me back to normal. He emphasised that there is still a lot of grey area around the subject and that there is no miracle cure. He mentioned getting me back to work many times, which I found curious and amusing seeing as I couldn't even sit through an episode of Kojak without feeling like rubbish. Anyway, he mentioned GET (Graded Exercise Therapy) which is basically a case of very gradually doing a tiny bit more exercise every time. The downside is that it's easy to misjudge and over-exert, putting you back in bed.

Now I loosely have a routine. I get up at 7am with my wife, take my meds and assess my body. It's quite a tricky thing to explain as there are no gauges, no bases of comparison. I gently try moving around, flexing and relaxing joints and muscles, all the while monitoring how tired I feel. Sometimes it's very deep rooted and I can tell straight away that I won't be doing much; other times I feel more free and light so can consider activities. At this point I want to take care to point out that, whilst I'm not having the time of my life, I am still lucky. There are plenty of people who are struck much crueller blows by ME/ CFS; some people are purely bed-bound - as in bed baths, catheters, etc. Some people cannot bear light or sound either so they lie in a dark and quiet room. They can't feed themselves, they can't play video games or watch telly, they just feel terrible. I don't like bright lights but I'm not that sensitive to them. I do find on the tired days I generally have a flu-like feeling where all you want to do is lie down and you hope to either fall asleep or stop feeling like rubbish.

Right now...

As I type this last paragraph it's around 9 o'clock on a Wednesday morning, March 2014. My wife is at work and I'm on the bed with my best friend by my side. Marmite is my little girl, she's a kind of spaniel/ collie cross, but there are other breeds involved somewhere I expect. Like most dogs, she is fiercely loyal and loves company. The other dog, Jack (collie/ retriever cross), is on guard patrol down stairs. I'm feeling quite good today; I've eaten a healthy breakfast and, despite aches, am considering doing any three of the following: doing the dishes, taking the dogs out, hoovering downstairs, doing some laundry, preparing dinner, playing Xbox. I'm using GET and pacing myself so it'll be on a work/ rest cycle. On days like today I can manage, I'm happy and fancy the challenge. I miss the old times and my old body but on the plus side, I have been able to use my time reaching out to people over Twitter, empathising, listening, and learning. The support network is phenomenal; you only need to be honest and friendly.

I'm going to finish now, and I'd like to say a massive thanks to my wife and friends; their support and love has been overwhelming at times, and that if you or someone you know has ME/ CFS please remember that there are many of us out there and we all want to help, so just find us.

xxxxx

To my friends new, my fellow sufferers,

Without ME I wouldn't have met you. I wouldn't have known your courage, your strength, your companionship. Suffering alongside each other, some grumbling, some not, but all with dignity and justification. Always there to give that ear to hear, that shoulder of support, as weak as it may be physically but a solid ledge to others.

Always ready to have a laugh at yourselves and then wanting to share, ready to praise the little achievements of each other, knowing how huge they really are. Understanding symptoms, the misery, and the frustration of living with this illness. The isolation, the loneliness, the unhappiness. Yet all quietly enduring your own gruelling days.

You put up with my despairing messages, texts of terror and heartache. You listened to my rants and tears. You let me vent it all and will do so again I am sure. I needed you and you were there for me, and are still.

A fellowship brought together by mutual ailments, international, most who we shall never meet in the flesh but do not need to. An online, electronic community, one of many faces, pale and pained, but smiling through it all.

Xx

To my fellow MEEPS,

I just want to say thank you. Never have I come across a group of people who suffer so much, who fight so hard just to keep going, yet are so supportive to others. I know it's not always easy; we all get tetchy and stressed at times because of all we're enduring, and our cognitive impairments can make misunderstandings happen all too frequently. However, the number of times I have seen people reach out to others with kind words, virtual hugs and practical tips is truly wonderful. I know that when I'm having a bad day there are places I can go to online where people will understand what I'm going through and will encourage me to keep going. When I have questions about symptom management or just coping day-to-day with this horrible disease, someone will have a suggestion. And on days when I've achieved something that the outside world would see as trivial, my fellow MEEPS will cheer me on and recognise what a big achievement it is to have my hair washed or whatever. It means so much to me, more than I can express. I don't know what I'd do without the online friends and support that expand my world beyond these four walls.

So thank you all. You are an amazing bunch of brave but hidden warriors who fight to climb your own versions of Everest daily just to survive, just to do tiny things like eating and washing that other people take for granted. Your countless battles may be unseen and unheard but you are not alone; there are others out there who understand and know what it's like to be living with this ****** disease. Hang in there. There is purpose in your life; you've already made a difference to me, just by being there and letting me know I'm not alone. Keep searching for smiles and laughter and beauty; don't give up. And keep reaching out to others, because together we are stronger.

Xxx

From me to other sufferers of ME,

I know how much it hurts you
When life is so very cruel
I know how much it pains you
When you can't go to work or school

I know that it's never ending
From head to toe and between
I know you're trapped in deep shadows
And light within the darkness is a dream

I know about the symptoms
Countless every day
Varying in level, yes
But always there to stay

I know about the suffering
When it feels like it just won't end
How it goes on and on and on
It seems only death may be your friend

I know about the indignities
Feeling a useless, burdenous thing
Being unable to lift a finger
Like a puppet on a broken string

I know about the endless problems
That take hours to merely list
I know about the snide remarks
And ignorant, 'is it REALLY as bad as THIS?!'

I know about the struggles
With the arrogant DWP!
Having to repeatedly prove you're slowly dying
Because they haven't a clue about ME!

I know about the disbelief
And barbaric treatment often deployed
For those without an advocate
It's sometimes impossible to avoid

I know about the prejudice
And name-calling still today
Even from our own friends and family
Who think us deliberately this way

I know about the loneliness
The isolation of a caged bird
I know about the guilt and sorrow
When you'd give anything to be heard

I know about the memories
That keep you sane and strong
Yet stuck in a time-loop of stillness
Longing to move up and on

I know about the hopelessness
That resides inside your heart
Covered by black clouds of rain
Praying for healing sunlight to start

But this is where you need hope the most
To get you through the years
To cope with all the horrendous trials
And wash away the flowing tears

For I know one day there will be a cure
With the right treatment, our lives will be turned about
We will eventually learn how to live again
Re-lit like flames that never fully burned out

© Emma Hodgson

Progressive ME sufferer of twenty years, since age eleven.

A message to those who suffer from one who has suffered,

    I know how you suffer. I know the torment, the despair, the fear. I know the symptoms, the unbelievable torture. Astounded at how my body can feel so ill. I have felt the shutdown of my mind, that ability called thinking. Such confusion. Lost in thoughts that race too fast to catch them, or run too slow to process them.

Times where I couldn't move, could barely breathe. Wrapped in pain. The terror of that moment, those moments, seemingly endless. Would I remain immovable forever? The uncertainty. Would I die this night? Will I recover? Will I walk again? What is this ME that savages my body, deletes my mind? So many questions. With no answer.

I've had to have help to sit and felt the room spin when I do. Had my head held up for me. I've had times of silence when I could not speak. The horror of not being able to communicate. And when I did have a voice, not having the words to describe. Who could understand, imagine this? I wouldn't unless I had been there.

For years feeling imprisoned not only in my room, but also in my body. Feeling the screaming panic as if buried alive. Fear of being tube-fed, hospitalised, being alive but as good as dead. An unmoving but breathing corpse. Never knowing how ill I could get, terrified of being unable to take my own life, too weak for that escape.

The fury towards the unbelievers, the desperation to be heard and recognised. The shame, the loss, the grief. Crying and crying and crying.

So I understand. As much as another can understand suffering who has been there.

But what I also want you to know is this... there can be change. Where I thought my legs would waste to nothing, I now walk. Where I thought my words would end, I speak. I can stand to look out of the window, am beginning to use my hands in craft again, I can think to write this. I can plan.

Yes, I still suffer but now I also hope. The fear has gone and I see brighter days before me. Before us.

There is a point to this life, a reason to continue.

Rest, relax, nurture your body and listen to its voice. Don't hate it for what it can't do, how it's let you down, put your life on hold. Give it nourishment, sympathy, time. You may be amazed at what can change.

So, you ME warriors, Boadicea and Braveheart, keep fighting, battle on, for one day you will succeed.

xxxxx

Thank you so much for taking the time to read this book.

Want to find out more about Invest in ME/ 'Let's do it for ME!' and the work that they do? Please follow the links for more information:

Invest in ME:

http://www.investinme.org

'Let's do it for ME!':

http://ldifme.org

Made in the USA
Charleston, SC
16 May 2014